Contents

Transcultural Geriatrics

Caring for elderly people of Indo-Asian origin

Partha Ghosh FRCP
Consultant Physician
Department of Elderly Care
Lister Hospital, Stevenage

Shahid Anis Khan FRCP
Consultant Physician
Department of Elderly Care
Lister Hospital, Stevenage

Radcliffe Publishing
Oxford • S

Radcliffe Publishing Ltd
18 Marcham Road
Abingdon
Oxon OX14 1AA
United Kingdom

www.radcliffe-oxford.com
Electronic catalogue and worldwide online ordering facility

British Library Cataloguing in Publication Data

A catalogue record for this book is available from the British Library

ISBN: 1 85775 745 9

Typeset by Action Publishing Technology Ltd, Gloucester
Printed and bound by T J International, Padstow, Cornwall

To my wife Asoka.
   Partha Ghosh

To my wife Nyla, without whose help and encouragement
this book would not have been possible.
   Shahid Anis Khan

Preface

Migration is as old as humanity itself. From the dawn of civilisation there have been links between the societies of the ancient world. As early as the first century of the Christian era, dynasties in the Indian subcontinent and the Hellenistic kingdom in Europe had begun to forge links. The invasion of the Indian subcontinent by conquerors such as Alexander and the creation of cities for their veteran soldiers and partisans led to closer cultural interaction. For hundreds of years trade links, warfare and improved maritime travel brought distant societies into close contact.

Migration is not new to the British. The great British tradition of travel and conquest along with their maritime superiority led Britons to far-off lands, acting as a catalyst for migration to the distant colonies. Over the last 100 years, the changing political milieu in Europe, as a result of the two great wars, and improved air travel have altered the shape of migration and laid the foundations for present-day British society. Though there are many different ethnic minorities living in our present multicultural society, Indo-Asians remain the single largest ethnic group in the UK.

The term 'Indo-Asian' refers to people who originated from the Indian subcontinent. The Indian subcontinent encompasses five countries, namely Bangladesh, India, Nepal, Pakistan and Sri Lanka. Some people of Indo-Asian heritage also migrated to the UK from former British colonies including East Africa, Fiji, the West Indies and South Africa. These people share with the British 250 years of history and have exerted a major influence on today's society.

Indo-Asians share many cultural values as well as their common geographical extraction. Yet they are a diverse group with many different languages, religions, customs and diet. There are many people in the UK who have little knowledge of Indo-Asians and the differences between the main ethnic groups.

Vast numbers of Indo-Asian immigrants who arrived in the UK in the early 1960s and 1970s are now retired or nearing retirement. There is a steady increase in the number of these elderly Asians, who thus have a profound impact on health resources and services across the country. Though many have adapted to their adopted country, they still have strong beliefs and preferences based upon their experience in their native country and culture.

Transcultural geriatrics is a relatively new branch of old-age medicine which explores the boundaries of sociocultural differences and their impact on human health. It is imperative that these differences are identified with sensitivity and needs are dealt with professionally. Failure to do so can have grave consequences for the patient and would result in wastage of precious resources. For healthcare workers, the task of delivering medical services to older people is unattainable if they lack insight into their sociocultural background and understanding of transcultural geriatrics.

Much has been achieved in the past three decades for the ethnic minorities living in the UK. Unfortunately, there is still little recognition of the needs of elderly people of Indo-Asian origin, i.e. those over 60 years of age. For the first time this population has exceeded the 500 000 mark. However, there remain major deficiencies in the recognition of their needs and in the provision of services. The needs of these elderly people not only affect them in isolation but could place an overwhelming burden on their families, friends and carers.

We wrote this book not only as professionals with experience of practising medicine in the Indian subcontinent and the UK but also as members of the Indo-Asian community living in the UK. This book is aimed at people who intend to expand their horizon of transcultural medicine. It is designed as a resource for professionals who wish to be better informed about their patients or clients. Doctors, nurses, paramedics, social workers, health planners, medical students, carers and politicians would find this text invaluable in all aspects of dealing with the elderly of Indo-Asian origin.

The resources and referenced literature in this book will not only be of interest to those involved in the care of Indo-Asian elders in the UK but will be invaluable to all countries where there is a growing elderly Indo-Asian population. Wider knowledge of medical, cultural and social interactions will inevitably lead to a clearer understanding of these patients' needs and thence to improved care.

Partha Ghosh and
Shahid Anis Khan
May 2005

About the authors

Dr Partha Ghosh. After graduating in India in 1971, Partha came to the UK in 1972 to further his training in geriatric and general internal medication – this was done in Shrewsbury, Ipswich and Birkenhead. Senior Registrar training was done in St Stephens, St Mary Abbott and Westminster Hospitals, London. He also studied tropical medicine at The Liverpool University in 1975.

In 1985 Partha was appointed Consultant Physician in Geriatric Medicine at Lister Hospital, Stevenage. He has been Clinical Director of Elderly Care Services and Associate Medical Director of the Trust and, since 1994, has been the lead physician for stroke services.

He has published more than 30 papers and is currently the editor (geriatric section) of the *Hertfordshire Journal of Medicine.* He is also an examiner of the MRCP Diploma and the Diploma in Geriatric Medicine for the Royal College of Physicians.

Dr Shahid Anis Khan is a geriatrician and general physician at Lister Hospital, Stevenage. He graduated from Allama Iqbal Medical College, Lahore, Pakistan in 1982. Shahid did his Senior Registrar training in medicine and elderly care at the West Middlesex University Hospital, Isleworth and at Charing Cross Hospital, London.

He served as Honorary Secretary for the North West Thames British Geriatrics Society and is presently North West Thames Representative on the British Geriatrics Society English Council. He is Clinical Tutor at Lister Hospital and an examiner for Royal College of Physicians for the MRCP Diploma and the Diploma in Geriatric Medicine. He has written more than 50 articles in medical journals and is editor of the *Hertfordshire Journal of Medicine.*

Acknowledgements

We are most grateful to Nyla Khan for reading through the manuscript and for her perceptive comments. We are grateful to Liz Hynard for helping with the manuscript and for her efforts in getting this book published.

Our sincere thanks also to the Librarian at the Lister Hospital Medical Library who was always very helpful.

Chapter 1

Transcultural geriatrics and the Indo-Asians: an international perspective

With rapid developments in clinical medicine and improvements in the social sector, the world's elderly population is growing at an astronomical rate. The current rate of growth of 2.4% per year is considerably higher than the world's total population growth. By the year 2025, 12% of the world's population will be aged over 60 years and 70% of them will live in developing countries. Most of this growth is expected in Asia, Africa and Latin America.

Ageing in the developed world

The ageing population in developed countries has increased gradually over the last 100 years, mostly as a result of improved socio-economic conditions. In the later part of the 20th century, the elderly population increased more rapidly and is still rising. In some European countries the elderly population has already exceeded the 20% mark and by 2050, one in three Europeans will be aged over 60. Elderly people tend to have greater health and social needs, as seen in the UK where people of 65 years and over now occupy two-thirds of general and acute hospital beds.

Ageing in the developing world

Many developing nations are experiencing the phenomenon of mass ageing for the first time, with some societies ageing more quickly than others. By the year 2025, 70% of the world's elderly population will live in developing countries. In some Asian countries the increase in the elderly population could be up to 400% over the next 25 years. It took over 100 years for Belgium's population aged over 60 to increase from 9% to 18% but Singapore will achieve this doubling in just 20 years. Similar trends are predicted for many South East Asian countries which will result in the emergence of new disease patterns, increasing chronic disability and changing social norms.

Reliable demographic data from the Indian subcontinent are not readily available. Like most developing countries, life expectancy has increased in this part of the world. Life expectancy at birth in India has risen considerably over the past three decades and is still rising. From 53 years in 1975, life expectancy reached 64 years by the year 2000 and is expected to be 72 years by the year 2025. India's next-door neighbour Pakistan has shown similar trends with respective figures of 53 years, 66 years and 74 years. By the year 2025, out of the 11 largest populations of elderly people in the world, India, Pakistan and Bangladesh will be the three main countries. India alone will have 150 million people over the age of 60 years.

There is a close association between ageing and chronic disease. However, in many developing countries the concept of chronic disease requiring long-term treatment for health preservation is not developed. Globally there are indicators that chronic disease will form a much higher share of overall disease and most of this burden will fall on developing countries. This has implications for health planners, economists, the sociopolitical framework of society and the private health sector. In less developed countries where resources are scarce, a partnership between patients and health service providers would be of paramount importance for an effective health system, as highlighted in the recent World Health Organization reports.

Traditionally families have looked after their elderly relatives in many developing countries. Though it is envisaged that in the short term these family values would continue, with the worldwide trend of declining birth rates, nuclear families, emancipation of women and increased migration for jobs, communities would replace the role of extended families. With the paucity of state-funded services for older people, the private and voluntary sectors would play a major role in delivering these services.

According to the International Organization for Migration, there has been acceleration in worldwide migration. In just two decades worldwide migration has doubled. In 1975 the total number of migrants worldwide was 84 million and this increased to 175 million in year 2000. The predicted number of international migrants for the year 2050 is 230 million. At present the UK has a policy of encouraging permanent immigration with the expectation of accommodating 150 000 migrants a year.

The trends in international migration and mass ageing in developing countries, especially the Indian subcontinent, will affect the healthcare systems of Western countries including the UK. There would be more elders of Indo-Asian background coming to the UK either as migrants or asylum seekers. There would be some who would accompany permanent migrants as their parents and some would be visitors and tourists. These changes will have a significant impact on the growing Indo-Asian population and will inadvertently affect the health services.

Definition of old age

There is no universally agreed definition of old age. The spectrum of disease starts to change and disability rises after the age of 60 years. Older people are not a uniform group and they have a broad range of needs. For service development, they could be separated into three main groups.

First, there are the *young elders*, those people who have just retired, i.e. aged between 55 and 65 years. They are generally well and are active. The goal for elderly care services is to extend disease-free active years.

The *transitional group* is in transition between healthy active life and frailty. This transition occurs between 65 and 80 years. The goal for health planners is to identify emerging problems, prevent disease and reduce long-term dependency.

Frail older patients are generally over 80 years of age. They merit special attention as they have a significantly higher level of pathology, chronic disease and disability which requires specialist services, skills and higher resources. The goal is to recognise the complex interactions of physical, mental and social issues and to provide a service which meets the needs of these patients and their carers. In some countries this group of very old people is growing faster than the rest of the elderly population.

Transcultural geriatrics

The medicine of old age is commonly called geriatrics. It is the branch of general medicine concerned with the clinical, rehabilitative, preventive and social aspects of illness in middle age and beyond. Transcultural geriatrics is the branch of old-age medicine that explores the boundaries of sociocultural differences and their impact on human health.

On one hand, there is a different pattern of disease presentation in the later stages of life along with slower response to treatment. On the other hand, the combination of multiple pathology, chronic illness and old age makes predicting the course of illness much harder. High morbidity with chronic disease and increased multidisciplinary rehabilitation needs support the call for specialist skills. The ethos is to help restore an ill, disabled person to the level of maximum ability. Hence a comprehensive service for elderly patients would need specialist departments to meet all healthcare needs.

In many developed countries the evolution of medical services for older people has resulted in different models of service deliveries. All these models share the common goal of ensuring that elderly patients have access to the skills and experience of a physician in elderly care medicine and the specialist services of the multidisciplinary team. The local needs of the community and the location of the department influences the development of services on a specific model. The traditional 'needs-related' model of care is more suitable for a service that is based at a non-acute site, whereas the 'age-related' model has long been favoured by many district general hospitals in the UK.

The 'integrated model' has been the most favoured model of care. It is currently practised in most hospitals in the UK where, undoubtedly, old-age medicine is best developed. The service provided by an individual organisation may need to consider a combination of models or variations but the type of service must meet all the needs of elderly patients.

Disease prevention is an integral part of elderly care medicine. To extend an active and healthy lifestyle is the biggest challenge for all involved with the health needs of the elderly population. Lifestyle changes to decrease cardiovascular risks, the benefits of physical activity with multifactorial intervention to decrease falls and nutritional support to maintain independence are but a few key areas. Vaccination, prevention of osteoporosis and thromboprophylaxis for thromboembolic diseases are some of the other areas in need of attention. Strategies to further enhance and consolidate these services have been targeted in the National Service Framework for Older People for England and Wales. The

UK government has set excellent standards and milestones for development on various aspects of health provision in the National Service Framework for Older People and the Health Improvement Programme (HImP).

End-of-life care is an integral part of a comprehensive elderly care service. This aspect of treatment has been provided in the developed world on the principles of diagnosis rather than need. There are lessons to be learnt from the pitfalls of such a system which leaves many terminally ill patients without specialist care. The model most suitable for palliative care would be one that prioritises resources on the basis of need rather than diagnosis.

In many developing countries, end-of-life care is influenced not only by health resources and expertise in this field but also by local customs, religious beliefs and social practices. Issues at this stage of life need to be thrashed out by open debate and addressing the needs of the community. Rights of dying people, delaying death or undue hastening of death and support for carers are just a handful of issues which serve as stepping stones to a much wider debate.

The future

The challenge for the developed world is to adopt a community-oriented approach and provide the highest attainable quality of health for older people. Recognising cultural and gender differences in old age with a pledge to ensure the same access to heath and social needs for all elderly people would be essential. Developed nations should share and disseminate the wealth of knowledge and expertise on age and ageing which they have acquired over the last 50 years with the developing countries.

Developed nations will have to accept migration as a fact of life which needs appropriate management rather than opposition. This phenomenon has continued for centuries and has waxed and waned depending upon international politics and sociopolitical factors. There are gains to be achieved for all with proper and structured programmes for integrating migrants from developing nations.

The challenge for developing countries is to adopt a cohesive strategy for dealing with the problems of the changing demographic process, increasing burden of chronic disease and limited resources. Good health in old age is dependent upon interventions at an early stage in life. The message of 'healthy ageing' and decreasing premature disability needs to be at the heart of health promotion programmes in all developing nations. There is substantial knowledge about managing old age in developed countries which could in part be adopted to suit the needs of individual communities and could act as a foundation to better health in old age. Without timely provision for the growing elderly population across the globe, the whole health and social system is at risk of meltdown. The patients, policy makers and service providers should join forces with international bodies to tackle the growing challenges before the eruption of this demographic time bomb.

Further reading

Department of Health (2001) *National Service Framework for Older People*. Department of Health, London.

Greengross S, Murphy E, Quam L, Rochon P and Smith R (1997) Ageing: a subject that must be at the top of world agenda. *BMJ*. **315**: 1029–30.

Hobbs F and Damon B (1996) 65+ in the United States. In: *Current Population Reports*. US Bureau of the Census, Washington, DC.

International Organization for Migration (2003) *World migration 2003: managing migration. Challenges and responses for people on the move*. Report, United Nations Publications, New York.

Kessing R M, Strathern A (1998) *Cultural Anthropology: contemporary perspective*. Harcourt Brace, London.

Kinsella K, Taeuber C (1993) *An Ageing World. II. International Population Reports P95/92–3*. US Department of Commerce, Bureau of the Censu, Washington, DC.

Murray SA, Boyd K, Kendall M, Worth A, Benton TF and Clause H (2002) Dying of lung cancer or cardiac failure: prospective qualitative interview study of patients and their carers in the community. *BMJ*. **325**: 929–32.

Swart L, Dick J (2002) Managing chronic disease in less developed countries. *BMJ*. **325**: 914–15.

United Nations (1995) *UN Population Prospectus 1995 Update*. United Nations, New York.

United Nations (1999) *World Population Prospects: The 1998 revision (medium variant projections)*. United Nations, New York.

World Health Organization (2002) *Innovative Care for Chronic Conditions: building blocks for action*. WHO, Geneva.

Chapter 2

Historical perspective of immigration: the Indo-Asians abroad

In the second half of the last century the UK moved from being a virtually 'all white' Christian society to a multi-ethnic, multireligion, multicultural society. At the start of the 1960s only 0.25% of the total population of the UK were from the Indian subcontinent or Afro-Caribbean in origin. The 2001 census showed that 4% of the population was from the Indo-Asian communities, namely Indian (1.8%), Pakistani (1.3%), Bangladeshi (0.5%) and others (0.4%).

Who are the 'Indo-Asians'?

Before World War II people who came to the UK from the Indian subcontinent were called 'Indians'. The majority were either students or *lascars*, the seamen. In 1925, over 7500 'coloured' seamen at sea and ashore registered under the Alien Act of 1920. This figure was probably inaccurate as it included Indian, African and Arab seamen.

Lascars from the Indian subcontinent had been recruited since the 17th century. During the Napoleonic wars the recruitment of these seamen became more widespread. During the Second World War, Muslim *lascars* from Jullundar and Hoshiarpur (Punjab), Mirpur (Kashmir) and Sylhet (Bengal) laid the foundation of the present-day Indian community in the UK. Most of these seamen settled on a temporary basis in the dockland areas of London, Cardiff, Liverpool, South Shields and Glasgow. Some, particularly from Sylhet (now part of Bangladesh), started opening 'Indian' restaurants. Dean Mahomet had the dubious honour of opening the first Indian restaurant, named the 'Hindostan Coffee House', at Portman Square in London. Born in Patna, India, in 1759, he joined the East India Company at the age of 11 years and became a *subidar*. He came to Great Britain in 1784 to introduce the art of *champi* (head massage). Later, other Asian restaurants mushroomed and by 1940s there were 20 such restaurants in London.

The students came from predominantly middle-class Indian families to study law, economics, engineering, medicine and, the most coveted of all, the Indian civil service. Many of these students later became leading public figures. The most eminent of these were the three heads of the independent states after the partition of British India, namely Jawaharlal Nehru (India), Mohammed Ali Jinnah (Pakistan) and Solomon Bandarnayaka (Sri Lanka).

There were many other examples of 'influential' Indians in Great Britain. In the later part of the 19th century Queen Victoria had an Indian *munshi* by the name of Abdul Karim who would have influenced the Queen's perception of Indian affairs. Other eminent examples include British MPs Dadabhai Naoroji

(1892–5) and M Bhowagree (1895–1905). There were also a handful of assorted princes, *ayahs* (nannies) and peddlers who constituted the early Indian community.

Definition

The partition of British India in 1947 created an independent India, East and West Pakistan. Ceylon (Sri Lanka) and Nepal soon followed. East Pakistan became Bangladesh in 1972. The creation of these states caused difficulties in defining people who originated from these regions. The generic definition of 'Indian' was not politically acceptable. The classification into Pakistani, Indian, Bangladeshi, Sri Lankan and Nepalese has been used to define people from the Indian subcontinent. This classification was adopted by the Office of Population Censuses and Surveys (OPCS) in the 1981 census for epidemiological purposes and is now widely used in ethnic monitoring.

There are several million people from the Indian subcontinent who lived in ex-British colonies such as the West Indies, Mauritius, Madagascar, Fiji, Singapore, East and South Africa. This group was difficult to define but after the expulsion of Ugandans of Indian origin in 1972, 'Ugandan Asians' was the phrase used by the press. 'Asians' became the general term for describing primary and secondary immigrants from the Indian subcontinent. In the USA, however, 'Asians' were immigrants from South East Asia, particularly Vietnam, Cambodia and the Philippines.

Currently, there is no universally agreed overall generic definition for the immigrant population who originally emigrated from the Indian subcontinent. Medical researchers have used several terms, including Asians, South Asians, Indians and Indo-Asians, to describe this cohort. The phrase 'Indo-Asian' is probably most suited to describe primary and secondary immigrants of Indian subcontinent origin to the UK.

The prehistoric period

The ancestors of the present population from the Indian subcontinent came from five racial groups. The first group were the Aryans who came from Central Asia and entered India through the passes in the Himalayas. The second group were the Dravidians who occupied most of Southern India. The third group were Mongols who invaded from the north east and were mostly from China, Tibet and Myanmar. The fourth group were the Austrics whose origin is not known but the Austric languages are spoken in South East Asia and Australia. The last group were the Negritos who could have originated from Eastern Africa. Some primitive tribes who descended from this group still live in the Andaman Islands.

About 4500 years ago, in the Bronze Age, the Aryan civilisation flourished in the Indus valley and the evidence for this exists today. The ruins of Harappa on the banks of the River Ravi, south of Lahore, and Mohenjodaro on the banks of the River Indus bear testimony to this period. The Persian and later the Greek invaders called the Aryans 'Hindus' after the River Sindhu, now known as the River Indus.

From the Punjab, this civilisation flowed south and spread throughout the east. Down on the Ganges plain the Aryans met the Dravidians. The Aryans imposed their culture, laws and Sanskrit language on the rest of India although they themselves underwent some modification to absorb the influence of other cultures.

The genetic mixing of indigenous groups and foreigners started in prehistoric times and continues to the present day. This has contributed to the rich and diverse canvas of today's Indian subcontinent.

The Hindu Buddhist period

During the time of Buddha (556–483 BC) the Persian kings Cyrus the Great followed by Darius I extended their empire and seized large parts of western India. Later, Alexander the Great invaded India and stayed from February 326 BC to October 325 BC. The most famous of ancient rulers was King Ashoka who came to the throne in 274 BC and ruled India from Kandhar in the west to Assam in the east. His conversion to Buddhism led to the spread of Buddhism from India to China, Sri Lanka and the islands of South East Asia.

The Muslim period (1483–1818 AD)

For over a thousand years India was ruled by various dynasties. It was divided into a mosaic of kingdoms with a complete absence of national solidarity and political unity. This was exploited by the neighbouring western states, in particular the Turks (Suljoks), Persians (Ghaznavadies and Ghories) and Afghans.

The Moghuls exerted a firm hold on India in the 15th century with Emperor Babur conquering the northern regions. His successors extended his empire until the whole country was under one rule. Several great Moghul kings ruled India over the next 200 years. The Muslim empire strengthened under the leadership of tolerant Moghuls like Humayun, Akbar, Jehangir and Shah Jahan but its decline started in the late 17th century in the reign of Emperor Aurangzaib. His religious ideology probably contributed to the Hindu uprising led by the Marathas from Maharashtra followed by Rajputs and Jats from north western India. Discontent among the Hindu majority was voiced by Sivaji who in 1674 established the state of Marathas. This was designated as the *Hindu Swarajya*, meaning a Hindu state. This laid the foundation of the racial and religious discord between Hindus and Muslims which culminated in 1947 in the partition of British India into Pakistan and India.

The British Raj (1818–1947 AD)

The Portuguese were the first Europeans to discover a sea route to India. In 1498 Vasco da Gama sailed from Lisbon, around Africa and arrived in India. Subsequently Portuguese generals and viceroys arrived to establish their control over the spice trade to Europe. In 1510 Goa became the capital of the Portuguese domain and remained under its control until 1952.

In 1600 English merchants formed the East India Company for trade with India and soon were granted a charter by Queen Elizabeth I. In 1606, Sir Thomas Roe was sent as an ambassador of King James I to Emperor Jehangir's court. Over the next 100 years the British not only traded with India but also established a foothold while the Moghuls and the Hindu kings fought among themselves. In 1707 Emperor Aurangzaib's death started the disintegration of the Moghul empire. In 1717 English traders obtained a *firman* or a decree from the Nawab of Bengal to establish a permanent trading post in Calcutta for a small annual payment. The French were also keen to establish their influence and in 1674 Pondicherry was founded and soon after a settlement was established at Chandernagar near Calcutta.

By 1818 British rule was firmly established in India. Changes were being introduced to influence the ideology of the Indian people. Introducing Christianity and bringing changes to the social class, the caste system and ancient rituals like *sati* began in earnest. 'The white man's burden' had to be redeemed. Legislation to abolish slavery was passed and within a year another law was enforced which prevented landings of slaves in British colonies. Between 1808 and 1830 the slave population in the British West Indies dropped from 800 000 to 650 000. Ten thousand new replacements were needed immediately. This shortfall in labour could only be met by the export of the lowest layer of the labour force from India – the 'hill coolies' or the load-bearers.

India in the 1920s was a very conservative society. The East India Company recruited upper-caste Brahmans and Rajputs into the army. For the sugar and indigo plantations, workers of lower castes were recruited from the eastern states such as Bengal, Orissa and Bihar. They were not good workers and belonged to a semi-aboriginal society. They came down to the plains from the hills and would hire out their labour to the agricultural industry where they came in contact with British indigo farmers. These hill coolies were soon being lured by recruiting agents of British merchants into ships bound for the British colonies. The recruiters were known as *'araketia'* by the local people. No clear records were kept but it is estimated that between the 1840s and 1850s, nearly half of the labour force exported to the colonies consisted of hill coolies. Other recruiting districts were the Northern Indian State of the United Provinces. The embarking port of these 'coolie ships' was Calcutta, from where the indentured labourers would arrive in Mauritius with their final destination being the West Indies. Apart from coolies, there were refuse collectors, rickshaw pullers, farm labourers and other menial workers who were transported to British colonies in the West Indies, Africa, South East Asia, Fiji and Mauritius.

Ron Ramden's monograph entitled 'The Other Middle Passage' describes Captain Swinton's journey from Calcutta to Trinidad in 1858. This is one of the very first accounts of the plight of the coolies and life on board the ship *Salsette* which left Calcutta 17 March 1858 with 324 Indian immigrants, mostly from the hill district of Chota Nagpur. The ship's surgeon, Superintendent Dr John Dyer, had to deal with deadly infections like cholera, dysentery, diarrhoea and depression which led to hunger strikes. Psychological problems were compounded by the cramped conditions, seasickness, homesickness and death of friends and family on board. The voyage lasted 108 days and ended on 2 July 1858. The death rate among immigrants was high and 124 perished during the journey. Every death meant a loss of £13 and, in total, £1500 of potential revenue was lost. This sparked allegations and counter allegations between the Trinidad Harbour Master, the Agent General of Immigration, the Inspector of Health of Shipping and the Immigration Agent at Calcutta. On the face of it there were official concerns about the fatalities on board but the main reason was economic rather than the plight of immigrants. Those who were lucky enough to survive the journey had to face years of hardship on the plantations.

British immigration policies

The 1905 Alien Act was the first legislation to limit entry to the UK following the arrival of a large number of Jewish migrants from Eastern Europe. The start of World War I raised concerns of further immigration and the Alien Restriction Act of 1914 was introduced. After the war the Alien Act of 1919 followed by the Alien Order of 1920 allowed immigration officers to refuse entry to 'coloured' seamen who could not prove that they were British subjects. Other legislation, including the Special Restriction (Coloured Seamen) Order of 1925 and the National Identity Card of 1943, was introduced. As a result, as recently as 1939, the population of permanent 'Asians' and 'blacks' living in the UK was only 7000.

The Commonwealth Immigration Act of 1962 was created to restrict the settlement in the UK of 'coloured' British subjects from the Indian subcontinent and from the colonies who did not have job vouchers or special skills. This Act was intended to curb mass 'coloured' immigration and laid the foundations of a multicultural Britain. The Act was announced in October 1961 and the beginning of its implementation was July 1962 so during the intervening nine months there was a 'beat the ban' rush of immigration. This was fuelled by travel agents from the emigration zones and helped by cheaper means of travel. Labour requirements in the service sector (transport, railways and the National Health Service), plus demand in traditional industries such as cotton mills and foundries, fuelled the mass migration. Between July 1960 and June 1962 approximately a quarter of a million immigrants arrived in the UK. The Act also encouraged those who had originally intended to stay temporarily, and send money home, to settle permanently and later bring their families. Significant numbers of Sikh families arrived before the Act became a law while fewer Mirpuri and Kashmiri families availed themselves of this opportunity. Notably, very few Sylheti wives or children came to the UK. Before the Act the Indo-Asian population in the UK was predominantly male and the reunification of families ensured the future growth of this community. In the White Paper of August 1965 severe restrictions were introduced on dependents over 16 years of age. This became law by the Immigration Appeal Act of 1969.

Vouchers or job offers were given to doctors, dentists and other professionals. The respective professional bodies had responsibility to authorise professional qualifications. These skilled professionals were then sent to places where there were recruiting problems like the midlands, the north-east, Wales and Scotland. Most of the Indo-Asian doctors came to the UK only to acquire postgraduate qualifications but many stayed and went into general practice or became consultants in Cinderella specialties such as geriatric medicine, psychiatry, learning disabilities, etc.

East African Asians

British East African colonies gained independence in the 1960s: Tanganyika in 1961, Uganda in 1962 and Kenya in 1963. East African Indo-Asians who originated from Gujrat, Punjab and Goa were merchant traders, civil servants and artisans and were faced with the choice of opting for local or British citizenship. A significant number chose British citizenship as insurance, with the view of leaving the newly independent countries if the political situation worsened.

Kenya introduced its Immigration and Trade Licensing Act in 1967 and nationalisation and Africanisation began in earnest. British subjects from East Africa of Indo-Asian origin were not restricted by the 1962 Act from entering the UK. By 1967, 10 000 East African Indo-Asians had done so. This was seen as a crisis and further immigration restrictions were hastily introduced. The second Commonwealth Immigration Act of 1968 was passed by Parliament in three days. This Act restricted all UK passport holders from entering the country unless they, a parent or grandparent had been born, adopted or naturalised in the UK. This legislation affected 200 000 people and rendered their passports worthless. As a concession, a voucher system was introduced at the rate of 1500 vouchers per year, thus allowing 5000 people to enter the UK.

The Immigration Act of 1971 became law on 1 January 1973. On the same day the UK joined the European Economic Community, thus removing the entry restrictions on 200 million Europeans without much public debate. The effect of the new law was to bring primary migration from the new commonwealth to a halt. As a concession the voucher scheme was doubled to 3000.

President Obote's Trade Act of 1969 and the Immigration Act of 1969 kindled the Ugandan exodus of 1972. This Act brought restriction in business opportunities for non-Africans, i.e. Indo-Asians, causing extreme insecurity. Idi Amin expelled Indo-Asians who were holders of British passports issued by the British High Commission of Uganda, at very short notice. This caused a major crisis and debate, led by the Conservative government of Edward Heath. Fewer than 29 000 people arrived and were helped by the Ugandan Resettlement Board to settle in cities where there were no major Indo-Asian settlements. This community was to make a major contribution to British society in the fields of commerce and industry over the next three decades.

The British Nationality Act of 1981 became law in 1983, bringing nationality and immigration legislation in line. For citizens of the British Dependent Territories, such as Hong Kong and the Falkland Islands, legislation was introduced which barred their entry into the UK. The British Nationality (Hong Kong) Act granted the right to enter the UK to a desirable select few. Others under the British Territories citizenship were to receive consular protection after 1999. These rules affected the majority of Chinese and a few Indo-Asian Hong Kong residents.

The future

The migration of Indo-Asians to the UK is an ongoing phenomenon and will probably continue for some time to come. Concerns over immigration and asylum seekers are high on the political agenda. There is a tendency for a knee-jerk response to issues relating to immigrants and it is not uncommon for health issues to be dragged into these debates.

There will be new acts and laws to streamline patterns of immigration. The tide of immigrants will bring with it new groups of Indo-Asians and inevitably more elders of Indo-Asian origin. Robust planning and awareness of the needs of the ethnic groups will be the key to securing a better future for the immigrants as well as the host society.

Further reading

Chand T (1969) *A Short History of the Indian People* (5e). Macmillian, Bombay.

Coker R (2004) Compulsory screening of immigrants for tuberculosis and HIV. *BMJ*. **328**: 298–300.

Jagan C (1994) *Forbidden Freedom – the story of British Guiana* (3e). Hansib Publications, London.

Ramden R (1994) *The Other Middle Passage. Journal of a voyage from Calcutta to Trinidad 1858*. Hansib Publications, London.

Spencer IRG (1997) *British Immigration Policy Since 1939. The making of multi-racial Britain*. Routledge, London.

Tinker H (1993) *A New System of Slavery – the export of Indian labour overseas 1830–1920*. Hansib Publications, London.

www.movinghere.org.uk

Chapter 3

Ethnicity and ethnic elders: the sociocultural background

In the decade to 2001, the ethnic minority population in the UK grew by 53%. This phenomenal increase in population (1991 to 2001) has been from 3.0 million to 4.6 million which accounts for 7.9% of the total population of the UK. Asians of Indian, Pakistani and Bangladeshi origin accounted for nearly 50% of ethnic minority groups. Another 15% of the ethnic population described their ethnic group as mixed. Hence people of Indo-Asian origin were the largest ethnic minority group in the UK with nearly 2.5 million people.

Box 3.1 Population of the UK broken down by age and sex	
All ages	58.8 million
Men 16–64, women 16–59	36.1 million
Men 65+, women 60+	10.8 million
Under 16	11.9 million

Society, customs and values are not constant entities but are constantly being modified by the winds of change. This transformation is influenced by politics and the economic climate as well as social fashions. Together they modify and redefine social boundaries. There is no universally acceptable definition of ethnicity and it is less likely that we would devise a universally agreed taxonomy. The term 'Asian' has loosely been used to describe all immigrants of Asian origin, which hides the rich diversity within the Asian community. Though there are subclassifications such as the one used by the Office of Population Censuses and Survey, 'Indo-Asians' in a broader sense covers the people of Indian subcontinent ancestry.

For the first time in the UK, the population aged over 60 has increased to 21% and the estimated numbers of the elderly of Indo-Asian origin exceed half a million. This is a pivotal point in the lives of these people as they are confronted with major changes. Their health needs are transforming along with the spectrum of disease as chronic disability increases. These ethnic elders are, however, not a uniform group and have a broad range of needs. There is noticeable variation in the elderly population within various ethnic groups, with a lower proportion of older people in Pakistani and Bangladeshi communities. On the whole, the population of elders of Indo-Asian origin is increasing rapidly and will mushroom over the next two decades. Unfortunately there is a dearth of information regarding most aspects of their lives. Social policies pertaining to Indo-Asians elders are based on perceptions and assumptions with little evidence-based research.

Indo-Asian ethnic groups in the UK

The UK is a true multicultural society with a large Asian community. To many an untrained Western observer, Indo-Asians are distinguishable by the colour of their skin, their geographical location, clothes and language. Their sharing of these differences leads to a common misapprehension that they are all alike.

Most health professionals would find themselves ill prepared coming into contact with an elder of Indo-Asian background. They would be handicapped by a lack of knowledge about the different subcultures which exist within the Indo-Asian population. Their concepts of sickness, attitude to illness, expectations and emotional reactions to stress and disease are very different from those of Western patients and in some cases are unique to each specific subculture. The response to a medical problem could trigger unfamiliar and bizarre behaviour which could easily be misinterpreted as 'pathological' but might be quite rational and understandable in the light of the patient's religious and social beliefs, cultural practices or past experience.

All Indo-Asians are not the same just because they share certain physical similarities. In reality, many have very little in common and originate from areas thousands of miles apart. For example, a Pathan from Pakistan would have as much in common with a Tamil from Sri Lanka as a Finn with a Sicilian.

Different cultures and subcultures define their own boundaries for normality and how to deal with what they perceive as abnormal. Knowledge of these cultural differences is highly desirable and lacking this background information, health planners and health professionals may fail to either perceive a problem or find a satisfactory solution.

Indo-Asians are not a homogenous group. It is important to have an insight into the background of the immigrants with knowledge of their country of origin. Many pathologies have a social, geographical, cultural and genetic basis. Without an insight into the cultural background, some pathologies could be completely missed.

Over the past 40 years, the Indo-Asian community in the UK has gone through a rapid metamorphosis and in the process has made an impression on many aspects of British life. Some of these changes have been occult, others more obvious. Those most affected by change are the elders of Indo-Asian origin and as these changes are continuously modifying this group, they merit regular reviews.

The 2001 census showed that ethnic minority groups were more likely to live in England than in other parts of the UK. They constitute 9% of the total population in England as compared with 2% in Scotland and Wales and less than 1% in Northern Ireland.

In comparison with the 1991 census, the ethnic minority population in

England increased from 6% to 9% partly due to the addition of mixed ethnic groups in 2001. However, an increase in population has been recorded in every Indo-Asian ethnic group in England. Indians form the largest minority group, followed by Pakistanis, Bangladeshis and those of mixed ethnic background. Two per cent of the population of England and Wales are Indian, with Leicester having the highest proportion (25.7%). The second largest community is in the west midlands (13%) followed by the south east (8%). A high proportion of people of Pakistani origin reside in Yorkshire and around the Humber (2.9%) and the west midlands (2.9%).

Indo-Asians are by and large urban dwellers. Nearly 45% of all ethnic minority people live in London where they constitute 29% of all residents. In some London boroughs they make up a sizeable chunk of the population.

Geographical background

During the Raj era, the Punjab province of India had close associations with the British army as it provided the bulk of recruits, while the Bengal province provided seamen for the merchant navy. Some of these associations laid the foundations for the earliest immigration to the UK and, later on, some areas of the Indian subcontinent developed a strong tradition of migration.

The post-war era saw a sudden surge in a rather underprivileged Indo-Asian labour force arriving to work in British factories. They came by invitation in the 1950s and 1960s. The majority of these migrant workers came from rural farming communities, mostly from remote and economically underdeveloped areas where educational standards were low and healthcare was poor. These migrants brought with them strong traditions and values common to their rural communities. They resisted cultural change as their main aim was to improve their financial standing back home and most did not intend to settle permanently in the British Isles. They lived within their social groups and made little effort to learn local customs or improve their language skills other than what was essential to earn a living. These attitudes persisted to some extent even after they became settlers. Apart from other stresses of immigration these people had to deal with the transition from rural life to urban living.

This group was unique in several respects as they had left their motherland in their twenties and thirties. They had little education and many had little command of English. They arrived either alone or in small groups and later invited their spouses and children. The slow stream of economic migrants led to clusters of communities developing in the inner-city areas of industrial towns and cities. Their concentration was high in Birmingham, Bradford, Leeds, Leicester, Manchester, Coventry and London, where there is now a population explosion in the ethnic elderly population. Some invited their ageing parents from their countries of origin as they came to terms with their changing status from migrant workers to settlers.

The main ethnic groups who came from the Indian subcontinent included Bengalis from Bangladesh. They were mainly Muslim but those who immigrated from Indian West Bengal were predominantly Hindus. The Gujratis and Kutchis were mainly Hindu from Central, Southern and Northern India. The Sikh community came from the fertile plain of the Indian Punjab whereas

Muslim Punjabis belonged to Western Punjab, now part of Pakistan. The Mirpuris came from the Kashmir province of Pakistan and were Muslims. The Sri Lankan nationals were mostly Tamil and Sinhalese. Each of these geographical groups can be classified according to their language, customs, ethnic grouping or religious associations. Physical characteristics also differ a great deal from one part of the Indian subcontinent to the other.

The other main area of immigration was East Africa. Most of these people had immigrated to British East Africa in the 1930s but left for England in the 1970s due to the changing political scene. They belonged to the middle-class business community or were professionals. This group had a high literacy rate and enjoyed a good standard of living. They came from urban dwellings with a very different social background to the migrant workers from the Indian subcontinent. The stresses for this group were very different, as they had to cope with the horrors of forced migration and loss of possessions and wealth. They were from diverse ethnic and religious backgrounds with a strong majority of Gujrati Hindus. Many had family links with people already living in the UK and their ambition was not to return home but to settle in the UK. They invested in local businesses and adapted relatively quicker to the local language and to their adopted culture. This group has a higher proportion of elderly people as they immigrated as entire families with their dependents and elders. The arrival of other immigrants from East Africa led to the emergence of a strong business community. With the development of the food and retail business, the Indo-Asian community scattered throughout the British Isles.

A small proportion of Indo-Asian immigrants were from the professional classes, namely doctors, engineers and teachers who had come over for post-graduate education or for work and later settled permanently in the UK. This group was well educated and economically stable which was in sharp contrast to the majority of migrants of Indo-Asian origin.

The migration of Indo-Asians to the UK still continues. There is a constant trickle of older people entering the UK to join their children. This group faces different challenges from other groups of Indo-Asian elders, both on the socio-cultural front and in terms of the disease spectrum.

Social aspects of Indo-Asian life

Despite the differences, there are certain traits common to nearly every ethnic group of Indo-Asian origin. These traits are even stronger in the elders of these groups. In spite of living in the UK for decades, Indo-Asian elders still hold their cultural values dear. Though two-thirds of their lives may have been spent in the UK, they strongly associate with their country of origin. They are proud of their culture and heritage and most would try hard to preserve their cultural and religious identities, sometimes leading to conflict with the younger generation and with the general community.

The social fabric of society in the Indian subcontinent is woven on the framework of the extended family structure. The family is the nucleus of all activities and has a strong bearing on all its members who work together as a single unit. In most households there are three or four generations living under one roof. Age is considered a sign of experience and wisdom and hence the senior male elder of the family plays the lead role and acts as the figurehead of the family. He has the final say in all matters. In the absence of a senior male figurehead, the eldest female adopts this lead role. Parents, especially when old, are considered the responsibility of the children and are well looked after in their old age. Families share the burden of disease and old age and look after their near relatives and even help their neighbours. This is not only a social custom but in some groups a religious duty. Shying away from these responsibilities may make people lose face within their communities. The older members in all subcultures are equally respected and are given a high status. They are actively involved in social affairs and play a dynamic role in local politics.

The women in the Indian subcontinent work in all walks of life. In the villages they form an important part of the workforce and are the backbone of cottage industry. With the increase in literacy, females are now working in all sections of society. However, the earlier female immigrants to the UK were less likely to be educated or to have a vocation as they came with their families and mostly looked after the household and the children. Nonetheless they exerted a strong influence on their families. They not only had sole charge of running the household but also exerted control on the social activities of the family.

Languages

There is a rich diversity of languages in the Indian subcontinent and most Indian immigrants are multilingual, with the majority having a command of two or three local languages other than English. There are numerous dialects of each of the local languages and this changes from one geographical area to another. The main languages in the Indian subcontinent use three different alphabets and though there is similarity in some of the spoken languages, people may not be able to read or write others.

The principal language of immigrants from Pakistan is Urdu with Punjabi, Mirpuri and Pushtao as their local languages. Hindi, Punjabi, Gujrati, Kutchi, Marathi and Bengali are some of the leading languages spoken by migrants from India and the principal language of Bangladesh is Bengali. The immigrants from East Africa speak the language of their original area of migration in India but are also fluent in Swahili. English has been the official language of the Indian subcontinent and is widely spoken by the educated masses. It is worth noting that many elders from the ethnic communities never had any education and hence are not able to read or write in English. Some are even unable to write in their own languages but most would understand spoken English.

Age can have a significant impact on language. A majority of elders from ethnic minorities are multilingual. In old age, some elders from ethnic minorities may revert back to their primary language or languages even if they had a good command of English during their working life. This transition may be a gradual process and occurs over years. Certain disease processes can hasten this transition, as seen in patients with cognitive impairment or occasionally with depression. These patients usually revert back to their primary language or mother tongue. Rapid loss of multilingual capabilities is rare but can be seen in patients acutely after a stroke. In some a certain aspect of language may be lost, in others the ability to communicate in a given language could be completely wiped out. Writing abilities are also affected in many elders due to stroke, Parkinson's disease or severe arthropathy.

Religions

According to the 2001 census, less than 6% of people in the UK have a religious affiliation other than Christianity. Of these, Muslims make up 3%, Hindus 1% and Sikhs 0.5%. Overall, 3% of the population of England is Muslim, with 0.7% of the Welsh. Thus Muslims are the largest group after Christians in the country. The second largest group after Christians and Muslims are the Hindus, with 1.1% in England and 0.2% in Wales. Sikhs make up 0.7 % in England and 0.1% in Wales.

Box 3.2 The main religious groups in the UK (2001 census)

Christian	42 079 417
Muslim	1 591 126
Hindu	558 810
Sikh	336 149
Buddhist	151 816
Others	178 837
No religion/religion not stated	13 626 299

In the UK, London has the highest proportion of Muslims (8.5%). Nearly 36% of the Tower Hamlets population and 24% of the population in Newham is Muslim. Harrow has the highest proportion of Hindus (19.6%). Over 8% of the populations of Hounslow and Ealing are Sikh. The district with the highest proportion of Sikhs is Slough.

In the Indian subcontinent, religion exerts the strongest influence on all aspects of life. The main religions in the Indian subcontinent include Hinduism, Islam and Sikhism. Though people are divided into various religious groups, the zest for religion is common to all. Religion provides a template for living and is the most sensitive of all issues. It plays a pivotal role in social, political and family life in all subcultures. Religious teaching heavily influences every aspect of life, including attitudes to illness and medical intervention. Devoting one's life to one's religion is considered the ultimate goal and people judge themselves and others on the basis of their commitment to it.

All main religions have strict dietary restrictions. Deviating from these is considered a betrayal of faith and those who digress are looked down upon by their communities. A person consuming food prohibited in another religion could easily ignite strong religious sentiment and occasionally this leads to major riots. In the UK, most elderly migrants still adhere to their dietary restrictions even if they have to go without food.

Fasting is a part of all religions and should be considered when treating patients. During fasting, a patient may refuse to take medicine, which could raise concerns while treating patients with chronic conditions such as diabetes. It is worth remembering that Muslims are exempt from fasting during illness or long-distance travel.

Diet and food

Food has a special place in Indo-Asian cultures and dominates religious and cultural events. The significance of food as a healing agent in illness is deeply rooted in the Asian psyche. Some food products are considered more nutritious and are specially prepared at a time of illness. These products may be brought to hospitalised patients as part of the family's and friends' attempts to show their affection for the patient.

There are stark differences in the dietary practices of the various Indo-Asian minorities, mostly as a consequence of geographical, religious and cultural practices. Traditionally most Hindus are forbidden to consume food containing animal products. They believe in the interdependence of life and reincarnation. They are strict vegetarians and some factions would disallow fish, shellfish, eggs and even onions and garlic. The cow is considered sacred and its slaughter is forbidden in most states of India. Offering beef to a Hindu would cause severe offence.

Traditionally Muslims are very particular about food. They eat meat of selected non-carnivorous animals, provided a Muslim has conducted the killing in a ritual manner similar to the Jewish process of producing kosher meat. In Islam, the process of killing the animal is called *halal* and the meat is labelled *halal* meat. The process of *halal* is considered humane and drains blood from the carcase as consuming blood is prohibited. The process of producing *halal* meat is to some extent similar to kosher meat for Jews. Muslims are allowed to eat kosher meat if *halal* meat is not available. *Halal* also refers to the animals which are allowed for human consumption under the Muslim religion. Animals which are carnivorous or are scavengers are not allowed and hence are not considered *halal*. Muslims are very careful about pork as pigs are considered unclean because of their scavenging habits and hence its consumption is strictly forbidden. Pork placed next to other edibles would cause revulsion and many Muslims would not touch a tray of food if there were any suggestion of it being contaminated with pork products. They would refuse bread, biscuits or fish if lard had been used in its preparation. Pork on the whole is considered unclean and avoided by most groups in the Indian subcontinent. Similar attitudes to pork prevail among the elderly British Indo-Asian communities. Most Sikhs would eat meat but rarely eat beef and many would avoid pork. However, they would not eat *halal* or kosher meat. Some Sikhs are strict vegetarians.

Unfamiliar food and especially lack of knowledge about its ingredients could cause confusion to most elderly patient and, if uncertain about its ingredients, they may refuse to touch hospital food. Sea food and in particular fish meat is one product exempt from religious restrictions and consumed by nearly all religious groups, the exception being the strict vegetarians. A few sects avoid fish without scales and crayfish. Dairy products, pulses, rice, vegetables and chapattis made of wheat flour are the main components of diet for all areas.

The dietary habits of the Indo-Asian community have not been well studied. Dietary habits exert a major influence on risk factors such as obesity, diabetes and coronary heart disease. There is ample evidence that risks for cardiovascular disease can be reduced by a diet containing a high proportion of vegetables, oily fish, fruit and fibre. Over the past few decades energy consumption has gone down in Indo-Asian food. Similar trends have been observed in India as well.

Consumption of *ghee* (clarified butter) may play a part in the abnormal metabolic profile of insulin resistance syndrome so commonly observed in Indo-Asians. Increased consumption of *ghee* and raised levels of trans fatty acids and low linoleic acid in fatty tissue may have some bearing on the increased risk for coronary heart disease. There is clear evidence that consumption of *ghee* is atherogenic and should be discouraged; along with encouraging low saturated fat products, this may have a beneficial effect. However, the higher mortality from coronary heart disease in Indo-Asians cannot be explained only on the basis of diet. The diet of the Indo-Asian is carbohydrate rich and differs from the European diet. Hence the advice give to the white population to follow a high-carbohydrate diet will be ineffective. In the Indo-Asian population, restriction of calories and lowering of fat consumption may be more appropriate for patients with coronary heart disease or insulin resistance syndrome.

There are certain characteristic dietary patterns within the Indo-Asian communities living in the UK. Bangladeshis have the lowest consumption of fruit but the highest consumption of red meat and fats. Pakistanis have the lowest consumption of vegetables. Except for Pakistani men, all other groups have lower fruit consumption than women in their ethnic group. Salt consumption is high in all Indo-Asian foods.

Diet and disease

For centuries, illness in the Indian subcontinent has been treated by a change in diet. Many elderly Indo-Asians firmly believe that the root cause of illness is food and most patients or their relatives would make lengthy enquiries about dietary preferences. They would expect the doctor to know about and advise them of the products they should avoid and the ones they should specifically eat during their illness. Some would insist on knowing the precise drink for swallowing tablets, i.e. whether the pills should be taken with milk, tea or water.

There is no single definition for the Indo-Asian diet as the Indian subcontinent encompasses thousands of different social and cultural groups. There is little health-based research on the dietary contents of the regional variations but there has been no evidence to suggest that the diet is atherogenic. The total fat content of Indo-Asian diets is no different from that of the general white population in the West but the ratio of saturated to polyunsaturated fat is high.

The high risk for coronary heart disease in Indo-Asians may be in part linked to dietary factors although, as mentioned earlier, this could not be the sole reason.

Diet and obesity

For centuries being overweight was considered desirable in the Indian subcontinent. It was linked to prosperity and indicated good health in a society where chronic malnutrition was rife. It portrayed a person not affected by chronic disease such as tuberculosis. These values still dominate many elders of Indo-Asian origin who would consider being overweight desirable. Notably, weight and height decrease with age in Indo-Asian elders.

Overall, obesity is low in Indo-Asians as compared with the general British population but they have a higher fat content and more subcutaneous fat.

Indo-Asian men have low levels of obesity. However, the pattern differs as they have more central or visceral obesity which is an important predictor of diabetes and cardiovascular disease. Central obesity is also linked with glucose intolerance, hypertension, hypercholesterolaemia, hypertriglyceridaemia and low serum HDL cholesterol.

Body mass index (BMI)

The BMI is defined as weight in kilograms divided by height in metres squared (kg/m^2). The BMI cut-off point for obesity is 25–29 kg/m^2. It is a validated tool for measuring obesity or thinness and is easy to use. Increase in weight and BMI in adults is associated with increase in mortality and morbidity. The main limitation of BMI is that it is a proxy tool and cannot distinguish between muscle and fat.

Considerable controversy surrounds the use of the BMI in the Indo-Asian community. There is disparity between the European population and the Indo-Asians as the accepted level for obesity (BMI >30 kg/m^2) is lower for Indo-Asians. The result is that the BMI cut-off point for obesity will underestimate obesity-related risks in the Indo-Asian population. Asians as a whole have a lower BMI for the same age and have a higher percentage of body fat as compared with the white population. Ethnic-specific cut-off points for BMI are not generally used in Europe as they might cause confusion in multicultural European societies. There is no single cut-off point for all Asians but recently the World Health Organization has recommended a lower level of BMI as desirable for public health actions in Indo-Asians. A BMI of 23 kg/m^2 has been recommended as increased risk and 27 kg/m^2 as high risk.

Waist-to-hip ratio (WHR) is defined as the waist circumference in metres divided by the hip circumference in metres. Studies in India have shown a higher association between waist circumference and increased risks for glucose intolerance, diabetes and cardiovascular disease in South Asians as compared to Europeans. In the UK, obesity is higher in Pakistani women and lowest among Bangladeshi women.

Although central obesity is prevalent in both Indo-Asians and the native white population of the UK, it constitutes a greater independent risk factor for coronary heart disease (CHD) in the Indo-Asians residing in the UK. In the white population central obesity constitutes a risk for CHD in groups with glucose intolerance, hypertension and dyslipidaemia.

Malnutrition is not a major problem in Indo-Asian communities residing in the UK or Europe but may be a problem in some groups who migrate from third world countries to Europe.

Physical activity

Regular moderate exercise of 30 minutes a day has been shown to reduce cardiovascular risks. Lack of exercise is associated with obesity and increased risk of cardiovascular disease. It has been shown that Indo-Asians who are more active have a lower BMI and lower concentration of insulin and triglycerides.

The Asian population in the UK has a lower level of physical activity than the white population. According to the 1999 census, the proportion of Indo-Asian men participating in brisk walking was low: only 12–19% of Indo-Asian men as compared with 28% of the general population. Within the Indo-Asian community, Bangladeshi men were most likely to have a sedentary lifestyle. The figures for the female population were even worse, with only 10% of them engaging in brisk walking as compared with 22% of the general population.

Alcohol

Alcohol has been consumed in the Indian subcontinent since the dawn of time but it has never found wide cultural acceptance. Alcohol consumption is predominantly a male prerogative and is extremely rare in elderly females. Many Indo-Asian elders living in the UK would still strongly disapprove of it. As alcohol is an essential component of the Western lifestyle, it may lead to conflicts with certain groups of elders from ethnic minorities. These conflicts may be within the community or within families as the younger generations are far more tolerant of alcohol as a social drink.

Attitudes are now changing and some elders would accept alcohol consumption as part of a more Western approach. However, Muslims would disallow it and may even reject medicines containing alcohol. In general, British Indo-Asians are less likely to consume alcohol than the native population and those who do, consume smaller amounts than the general population.

Alcohol intake is associated with several medical and social problems, including cirrhosis, hypertension, ischaemic heart disease, violence and antisocial behaviour.

Table 3.1 Alcohol consumption in Indo-Asians in the UK (DoH 1999)

	Men	Women
Bangladeshi	4%	1%
Pakistani	9%	3%
Indian	67%	38%
General population	93%	88%

In the UK, 14% of Indian men drank above the recommended limit but less than 5% of men or women from Pakistani or Bangladeshi origin drank more than the recommended amounts. Two per cent of Indian women exceeded the recommended safe limit but the least likely to drink are Bangladeshi women. Overall, alcohol consumption decreases with age in Indo-Asians.

Smoking and tobacco use

Smoking is a major risk factor for cancer, stroke and coronary heart disease and exhibits a dose–disease relationship. It affects insulin resistance, glucose metabolism and haemostatic functions but these areas are less well described. Smoking is widespread in all Asian communities with the exception of Sikhs, for whom its use is prohibited by religion. Smoking is more common in elderly men than women but they are less likely to smoke heavily as compared with the general population. The prevalence of cigarette smoking decreases with age, the only exception being Bangladeshi men. However, smoking more than 10 cigarettes a day is more likely in Indo-Asian subjects with coronary heart disease.

Table 3.2 Self-reported cigarette smoking in British Indo-Asians (DoH 1999)

	Men	Women
Bangladeshi	44%	1%
Pakistani	26%	5%
Indian	23%	6%
General population	27%	27%

The results from the 2001 census showed that in the UK, 44% of Bangladeshi men smoke cigarettes. For Pakistani men, 26% smoked followed by 23% of Indian men. This is in contrast to 27% of men in the general population.

Cigarette smoking is exceeding rare in Indo-Asian women and those who do smoke are less likely to be heavy smokers. For the UK general population, men and women are equally likely to be smokers.

Smoking is strongly associated with a person's socio-economic class. Lower socio-economic classes are more likely to smoke, as seen in Bangladeshi men who were over-represented in the lowest socio-economic class.

Apart from cigarettes, there are other examples of tobacco smoking. One such habit is *huqqa* smoking, which is still common in some communities living in the UK. People may also smoke *biri*. Elders who smoke *huqqa* or *biri* may not admit to smoking if questioned regarding cigarette smoking.

Huqqa smoking

This is a form of tobacco smoking where a wooden or a plastic pipe is used with a metal or clay water reservoir acting as a filter. *Huqqa* smoking is an ancient tradition and a norm for men and women in the rural communities of the Indian subcontinent. Common in rural Indian and Pakistani communities, its use is rare in the urban middle classes.

Biri

Biri consists of rolled tobacco leaf which is smoked like a cigarette. It is a common method of smoking in the Indian subcontinent. Being relatively cheap, its use is common in the lower socio-economic group.

Chewing tobacco

Several forms of chewing tobacco are noted in the Indo-Asians.

Table 3.3 Use of chewing tobacco by Indo-Asian groups (DoH 1999)

	Men	Women
Bangladeshi	19%	26%
Pakistani	2%	2%
Indian	6%	2%

Paan

Paan or betel chewing is very common in many Asian countries and especially in the Indian subcontinent. It is allowed in all religions and social groups and is considered a recreational activity. The betel nuts are wrapped in betel leaf along with a concoction of limestone, catechu, herbs and other ingredients. *Paan* is chewed with or without tobacco paste (*zarda*) or without tobacco. The betel juice may be swallowed or spat out. Children as young as five are given *paan* with sweeteners wrapped in it, especially on religious or social occasions.

Though a part of social behaviour, *paan* chewing is a risk factor for many medical problems, namely carcinoma of the mouth and tongue and hepatocellular carcinoma. There is even the suggestion that it may predispose to stones in the kidney, bladder and gall bladder.

Several other forms of chewing tobacco are known in the Indo-Asian community including chewing plain tobacco and *paan masala* which is tobacco mixed with various ingredients. In the UK the highest consumption of chewable tobacco in *paan* is seen in Bangladeshi men (14%) and women (23%). Bangladeshi women have the highest incidence of chewing tobacco in one form or another. Tobacco is also popular among Bangladeshi men but they tend to use it in conjunction with cigarettes.

Old age

All over the world cultures vary in the way they perceive old age and the status they accord to older people. In the West, consumerism being the basic driving force, the elderly are seen as less productive and this leads to a decrease in social status with old age.

In the Indian subcontinent, old age is synonymous with wisdom. Elders are the guardians of history, tradition and culture. In the rural communities of the Indian subcontinent, old people are the sole source of history and they take a leading part in the traditional and ritualistic aspects of activities in their communities. Death of an elder may be seen as an irreparable loss to the community as pearls of wisdom may be lost forever.

Elderly people have a special place in Indo-Asian society. Elderly parents are the nucleus of the family and they have the final say in all domestic affairs. They are highly respected by their family and the community. Many older people give up work and major responsibilities after retirement. They expect the family to provide all the care they require, in sickness and in health. These traditional and social pressures may affect the use of social services, community care and provision for long-term care in nursing homes.

Age-related cognitive decline and mild cognitive impairment are not seen as a major health problem. There is a great deal of tolerance in these cultures and respect for old age does not vanish with the early signs of dementia. There is some evidence that Alzheimer's type dementia is less common and less severe in the Indian subcontinent. However, there is controversy over whether this is secondary to greater involvement of the elderly in the sociocultural fabric of society or due to shorter life expectancy.

Conclusion

The Patient's Charter specifically requires that cultural and religious beliefs of ethnic minorities be taken into consideration when formulating health policies. However, the elders of Indo-Asian origin not only face problems similar to the elders in the Caucasian population but also have increased risk of certain diseases. They are also exposed to racial discrimination and have poor access to health facilities. Language and social barriers, inappropriate housing and low income add further difficulties to these already disadvantaged communities. The only way of alleviating these disadvantages would be by better understanding of their culture, better training of health staff and a more sensitive environment.

Further reading

Community Relations Commission (1976) *A Guide to Asian Diets*. Social Services Section. Community Relations Commission, London.

Department for Education and Skills (2002) *Annual Local Area Labour Force Survey 2001/02*. Office for National Statistics, London.

Department of Health (1998) *Smoking Kills: a White Paper on tobacco*. The Stationery Office, London.

Department of Health (1999) *Saving Lives: our healthier nation*. The Stationery Office, London.

Department of Health (1999) The *Health of Minority Ethnic Groups. Health Survey for England*. Department of Health, London.

Dhawan J, Bray CL (1997) Asian Indians, coronary artery disease and physical exercise. *Heart*. **78**: 550–4.

Dhawan J, Bray CL, Warburton R, Ghambhir DS and Morris J (1994) Insulin resistance, high prevalence of diabetes, and cardiovascular risk in immigrant Asians. Genetic or environmental effect? *Br Heart J.* **72:** 413–21.

Eliasson B, Mero N, Taskinen MR and Smith U (1997) The insulin resistance syndrome and postprandial lipid intolerance in smokers. *Atherosclerosis.* **129:** 79–88.

Health Education Authority (1991) *Nutrition in Minority Ethnic Groups: Asians and Afro-Caribbeans in the United Kingdom.* Health Education Authority, London.

Health Education Authority (2000) *Black and Minority Ethnic Groups in England: the second health and lifestyles survey.* Health Education Authority, London.

Hedges BM, Jarvis MJ (1998) Cigarette smoking. In: P Prescott-Clarke, P Primatesta (eds) *Health Survey for England: the health of young people '95–97.* The Stationery Office, London.

Hill SE (1990) *More than Rice and Peas: guidelines to improve food provision for black and ethnic minorities in Britain.* The Food Commission, London.

Jacobson MS (1987) Cholesterol oxides in Indian ghee: possible cause of unexplained high risk of atherosclerosis in Indian immigrant populations. *Lancet.* **ii:** 656–8.

Jarvis M (1994) Gender differences in smoking cessation: real or myth? *Tobacco Control.* **3:** 324–8.

McKeigue PM, Marmot MG and Adelstein AM (1985) Diet and risk factors for coronary artery disease in Asians in northwest London. *Lancet.* **2:** 1060–90.

McKeigue PM, Shah B and Marmot MG (1991) Relation of central obesity and insulin resistance with high diabetes prevalence and cardiovascular risk in south Asians. *Lancet.* **337:** 382–6.

Miller GJ, Kotecha S, Wilkinson WH et al.(1988) Dietary and other characteristics relevant for coronary heart disease in men of Indian, West Indian and European descent in London. *Atherosclerosis.* **70:** 63–72.

Nath BS and Murthy R (1988) Cholesterol in Indian ghee. *Lancet.* **ii:** 39.

Paris P, Pogue J, Gerstein H et al.(1996) Risk factors for acute myocardial infarction in Indians: a case control study. *Lancet.* **348:** 358–63.

Pate RR, Pratt M, Blair SN et al. (1995) Physical activity and public health. A recommendation from the Centers for Disease Control and Prevention and the American College of Sports Medicine. *JAMA.* **273:** 402–7.

Ramachandran A, Snehalatha C, Latha E, Satavani K and Vijay V. (1998) Clustering of cardiovascular risk factors in urban Asian Indians. *Diabetes Care.* **21:** 967–71.

Reaven GM (1986) Role of insulin resistance in human disease. *Diabetes Metab Rev.* **1:** 143–7.

Rimm EG, Giovannucci FL, Willett WC et al. (1991) Prospective study of alcohol consumption and risk of coronary heart disease in men. *Lancet.* **338:** 464–8.

Smaje C (1995) *Health, 'Race' and Ethnicity.* King's Fund Institute, London.

Snehalatha C, Viswanathan V and Ramachandran A. (2003) Cutoff values for normal anthropometric variables in Asian Indian adults. *Diabetes Care.* **26:** 1380–4.

Wang J, Thornton JC, Russell M, Burastero S, Heymsfield S and Pierson RN Jr. (1994) Asians have lower body mass index (BMI) but higher percent body fat than do whites: comparisons of anthropometric measurements. *Am J Clin Nutr.* **60:** 23–8.

World Health Organization (1990) Diet, Nutrition and the Prevention of Chronic Diseases. WHO Technical Report Series 797. World Health Organization, Geneva.

World Health Organization (2004) Appropriate body-mass index for Asian population and its implications for policy and intervention strategies. WHO expert consultation. *Lancet.* **363**: 157–63.

Chapter 4

Indo-Asians: ethnicity and clinical practice

The provision of fundamental healthcare in a multicultural and multifaith society is a challenge facing many health services across the globe. Patients' cultural and religious beliefs have a profound effect on their health. Being aware of these perceptions is the first step in offering appropriate healthcare.

The way in which medicine is offered in the Western world is in a specific format of history taking and examination. Doctors and other health professionals focus on issues which they deem important based upon their training and experience. They may have different perceptions of patients from ethnic minorities and may subconsciously act with bias against a particular ethnic group. This brings them into conflict when treating patients from ethnic minorities whose perception of disease and treatment may be different from that of their health providers. This could fuel mistrust of Western medicine and lack of confidence in the doctor. Some may even have had negative experiences with medical services during the migration process and feel betrayed by the system. Their experience of prejudice may make them suspicious of anyone who might wield some authority over their health matters.

In a system where there may be a wide gulf between the patient and health professionals, it is imperative that efforts are made to bridge this gap by all means possible. Some basic understanding of difficulties with history taking and examination are described to help with the management of such patients.

History

There are some general aspects of history taking where cultural awareness may prevent frustration for the health professionals and undue anxiety for the patients.

Enquiring about the past medical history is a problem with many elderly patients. Previous written medical records may be useful and an occasional patient may put a large file of papers on the doctor's table, expecting him or her to find the relevant information. But in most cases the records will be incomplete or non-existent. Recent immigrants usually have little information regarding their health records. Despite undergoing major surgery in their country of origin, they may be totally unaware of the diagnosis. Families may be able to provide some information. Writing to hospitals and clinics in the Indian subcontinent is a futile exercise as very little information is retained and most records are kept by patients themselves.

One of the common questions asked by doctors or nurses is the patient's age or date of birth. This may cause difficulties, as many ethnic elders are uncertain about their exact age. Lack of education, ignorance and poor standards of record keeping in their country of origin contribute to this problem. In response to a question regarding their age, some may refer to a natural calamity, a national incident or occurrence in their country of origin which would be completely alien to a doctor in the UK. An approximate age is all one can achieve in many of these patients.

Certain questions in history taking may be perceived as threatening if the patients are unable to understand the reason behind the questions. The most common question which could be perceived as offensive is enquiry about their origin or duration of stay in the country. This is commonly interpreted as challenging their right to medical care or to be in the country. If it is explained before inquiring that the question is to explore the familial basis of pathology or geographical link to pathology, the conversation may be less threatening. This may even increase the patient's confidence in the doctor and will help in obtaining a more complete history.

In certain languages, for example Punjabi, words or diagnosis taken for granted in the West do not exist. Depression is a good example where the patient may stress physical more than psychological features. In some patients, emphasis on physical symptoms rather than psychological symptoms may be prominent because of the social taboos attached to psychiatric diagnosis. Body language may give more important information than words.

Reluctance of patients to answer certain questions is not uncommon. Some questions may be embarrassing especially if the doctor is of the opposite sex. Gynaecology, genitourinary medicine or bowel care are main areas where a health professional may encounter these difficulties. Reassuring patients and explaining the basis for asking questions helps in gathering appropriate information. Alternatively, getting a female health professional to deal with a female patient might prove more fruitful, especially while dealing with a shy elderly female.

Language difficulties are the biggest barrier to a good history. This may lead to problems between patients and their doctors as words may be misconstrued. Use of an interpreter is commonly recommended. This can be helpful but there is need for caution in using interpreters from the patient's own family. Help from a professional interpreter is ideal. Using a family member, especially a grandchild, may cause difficulties as the elders often do not like discussing intimate details in front of their grandchildren, especially if the interpreter is of the opposite sex. The patient may not wish medical details to be known to the interpreter or the interpreter may not express the true history and alter the symptoms in translation, based upon their own experience.

Even when a patient is able to converse in English, their understanding may not be adequate to express the subtleties of the language. Doctors and other health professionals should spend some time evaluating the patient's understanding of the clinical problem at the end of the consultation. This may save time in the long term.

Examination

Touch by a person of the opposite sex is not permitted in certain cultures. Muslim women may object to being touched by a male health professional.

Many elderly women from the Indian subcontinent would have reservations regarding an examination conducted by male nurses or doctors. Some Muslim men may also have inhibitions regarding touch by a female doctor. This is particularly so if the examination involves internal examination. After appropriate explanation, many patients would not object to touch for basic examination. However, based on cultural and religious beliefs, many would refuse intimate examination.

Every effort should be made to preserve the patient's modesty. A vast majority of ethnic elders have inhibitions about undressing for examination. This is part of their culture and would need to be considered by healthcare workers. Explanation regarding the importance of such examinations should be provided and only that part of the body exposed which is absolutely essential. Many elderly patients would be reluctant to undress in front of an examiner of the opposite sex. If possible, a doctor or a nurse of the same gender should conduct such examinations. If not possible, it may help to have an attendant of the same sex present at the time of examination. Some patients may refuse examination by a doctor of the opposite sex with the same ethnic background but may agree to the same examination by a doctor from a different ethnic background.

The difficulties of non-familiarity with dark skin are common in dealing with elders of ethnic origin. Many clinical signs may be missed if changes in the shades of skin are not accounted for. Pallor, jaundice and cyanosis are difficult to detect clinically with confidence in elderly patients. This could be very difficult in dark-skinned patients, especially when the signs are subtle.

Perception of health problems

In the Indian subcontinent, traditionally the emphasis is on cure of the illness. This is particularly the case for alternative medicine where treatment is given to eradicate the illness rather than to treat symptoms.

Many Indo-Asians have had treatment for illness in their countries of origin. In many cases the illnesses are short bouts of infection which subside over a short period of time. Even for more chronic illnesses, the treatment is predominantly of short duration and usually patients are prescribed a few doses of tablets or a series of injections. The reason for this is based on the fact that medicines are expensive and many patients are unable to afford them for a prolonged period. Hence long-term therapy for chronic illness is less common. In the West where chronic illness is rife, such experiences lead to poor drug compliance. This is a major health issue in many ethnic elders. Some may discontinue medications because of past experiences, others may stop them due to side effects or because they are unaware of their importance. The concept of prevention by medications is also an alien one for this generation. Taking tablets for the rest of their lives for a chronic pathology like dyslipidaemia is new to many elderly patients and promotes poor compliance with medication.

Patients who are vegetarian or have certain religious convictions would be offended if prescribed certain medications. This includes porcine insulin for Muslims and capsules with gelatine coating for vegetarians. When prescribing drugs, drug interaction with herbal medicine should also be considered. It is essential that the doctor spends time looking for any unexpected side effects.

There is usually reluctance on the patient's part to disclose use of alternative medicine to the doctor for the fear that it may cause offence.

Elders from the Indian subcontinent usually consider obesity as a sign of affluence and may not pay much attention to advice on losing weight. Repeated explanations may be needed to convince them to adhere to dietary or caloric restrictions.

In the Indian subcontinent, illnesses such as epilepsy, leprosy and tuberculosis have strong social taboos attached to them. Patients and families may try to hide such information even from the health professional. Explanation and reassurance may be required to acquire such sensitive information from the patient. Stroke may be considered a punishment from God and, for some, a chronic illness may be a retribution for their sins in this life. Negative attitudes to treatment and rehabilitation in such circumstances are very common. Sexually transmitted diseases or alcohol-related illnesses, though rare, may be a great cause for concern for many patients and their carers as they can bring shame to the family. Sensitivity and understanding would be vital if the patient is expected to revisit the health establishment.

Most elders of Indo-Asian origin will be aware of the diagnosis of cancer and will regard it as fatal. As the cancer services in their own countries of origin are underdeveloped, the outcome is usually poor and this reinforces their negative perception about cancer. Some may believe that cancer is contagious and would fear that they will become social outcasts in their communities after such a diagnosis.

Investigations

Ethnic elders generally avoid investigations, particularly haematological tests. This is again based on their experiences in their native land where the expense for such investigations is prohibitive. In some patients there may be a belief that giving blood for any reason is unhealthy. Muslim patients may refuse a blood test in the holy month of Ramadan between sunrise and sunset when they fast. They would also refuse any intravenous injections or drips during this month. Such treatments should be discussed in advance and in detail with the patient. If the medical problem is serious and requires urgent intervention, there are clear guidelines which exempt Muslims from fasting and under these circumstances transfusions or blood tests can be conducted. Awareness of these exemptions is important and this could also be applied to patients with a wide range of illnesses, including diabetes and asthma.

Investigations that may require samples of urine and faeces may cause difficulties with some elderly patients, as they believe they would be polluted by carrying such samples. There is good evidence to show that interventions in the community such as faecal occult blood monitoring have poor uptake by Indo-Asian elders. Acquiring such samples in the surgery or in the outpatient clinic may be more fruitful.

Principles of managing elderly patients

From the dawn of civilisation, the achievement of longevity has been one of humanity's greatest dreams. With improvements in medical science, this dream turned into an obsession. With the advent of new medications and the idea of combination of compounds, the dream is gradually turning into reality. As a result old age has become an important health and social issue in most developed countries.

The numbers of frail elderly people are increasing at an alarming rate and the numbers of elderly over 85 years of age are increasing even faster. Elderly patients occupy two-thirds of general and acute hospital beds in the UK. These patients differ from younger patients in many ways. Higher levels of pathology, chronic disease and disability are common in this group. There are complex interactions of physical, mental and social problems which make their management difficult.

There are certain principles of managing illness in old age which need special consideration when dealing with frail elderly patients (Box 4.1).

Box 4.1 Ten principles for the management of frail elderly patients

- Atypical presentation
- Late presentation
- Silent pathology
- Disease less symptom specific
- Symptoms less localised
- Impaired immunity
- Multiple pathology
- Polypharmacy and iatrogenic disease
- Presentation with geriatric giants
- Social presentation

Atypical presentations

Medical literature is generally based on experience with the younger population. For example, the average age for heart failure patient is 76 years but average age in the trials for heart failure is 63. Frail elderly patients may present to their doctors with generalised symptoms not specific for the presenting pathology. A fall is a common presentation in many elderly patients who have underlying infections.

Multiple pathology

Traditional medical teaching has been on the unitary disease model where each disease is taught on its own. However, in frail elderly patients it is the combination of several pathologies which makes the presentation complex and treatment more difficult.

Silent presentation

Disease may be devoid of its 'classic' symptoms, for example a patient presenting with painless myocardial infarction. However, true absence of symptoms is uncommon.

Late presentation

There are several reasons for late presentations in old age, of which confusion with symptoms of ageing, social isolation, atypical presentation and cognitive impairment are just a few. Fear of hospitalisation and institutionalisation may well be responsible for the delay in seeking help for medical issues. Poor vision and hearing complicate communication and accessibility to health services.

Geriatric giants

Immobility, instability (falls), intellectual impairment (confusion) and incontinence are the most common presenting features in elderly patients. These features can be a result of acute or chronic pathology and may overlap with features of ageing.

Impaired immunity

Infections are common in older patients. There are several reasons for the elderly to present with infections, including decreased efficiency of the immune system. The infections present with less specific symptoms and other features which may dominate presentation in younger patients, such as pyrexia, may be absent in frail elderly patients. Lack of inflammatory response in these patients may be another feature which complicates the clinical scenario and hence inflammatory markers cannot be relied upon to exclude infection when dealing with frail elderly patients. Impairment of the immune response may be a contributory factor for the high incidence of malignancy in older people.

Polypharmacy in the elderly

Fifty per cent of prescriptions are for those aged 65 years and over. Older patients benefit as much as the young from secondary and primary prevention treatment. Medications offer functional independence, improved quality of life and enhanced life expectancy. However, non-compliance with medications is common in older patients. This is the single most important reason for treatment failure and can be attributed to cognitive impairment, polypharmacy or poor knowledge of the disease and the medicine. Side effects of medication, for example urinary incontinence with diuretics, and social isolation may also play an important role in poor drug compliance.

Homeostasis

Impaired perception to change in the environmental temperature is not uncommon in frail elderly patients. This causes problems when there is a sudden change in temperature and can lead to either hypothermia in cold weather or dehydration in a hot climate. The problem is compounded by medications which may have an effect on the regulation of temperature or the body's home-ostasis, such as phenothiazines and diuretics.

Management considerations

Frail elderly patients make extensive use of medical and diagnostic facilities and have a longer length of hospital stay. They also require increased use of reha-bilitation and social service resources.

High-risk patients in the community

There are several groups of patients who would be classed as high risk if they have a combination of risk factors as detailed in Box 4.2.

Box 4.2 Issues which may alert health workers regarding high-risk elderly patients in the community

---

- Age over 80
- Living alone
- Bereaved/depressed
- Cognitive impairment
- Falls
- Malnourished
- Pressure sores
- Incontinent
- History of inability to cope in the past

More than 80% of those over 80 live independently in the community. Medical, psychiatric and social problems are interconnected and hence it is vital to take a multidisciplinary approach when dealing with frail elderly patients.

Recommendations

The issue of healthcare for ethnic elders is vast. The first step towards improve-ment in health for elders of Indo-Asian origin is awareness and cultural sensitivity in health professionals. Health professionals should be aware of the different ethnic communities in their area and their medical needs. They need to make an effort to learn a few basic aspects of their language and culture.

From the patients' point of view their communities would have to act and take giant leaps in bridging the gaps. Communication is the primary problem and it is tempting to suggest a blanket approach to improve communication. Nonetheless, patients come from diverse backgrounds and speak different languages. It is important that individual health issues are targeted in each ethnic group. Community leaders, politicians and religious leaders can play a major role and should be invited to join forces in delivering a better health service. Without a multifaceted strategy in dealing with diverse issues, it will be impossible to improve the health needs of elders from ethnic minorities.

Further reading

Eshiett MU-A and Perry EHO (2003) Migrants and health: a cultural dilemma. *Clin Med*. **3**: 229–231.

Helman CG (2001) *Culture, Health and Illness*. Arnold University Press, London.

Henley A and Schott J (1999) *Culture, Religion and Patient Care in a Multi-Ethnic Society*. Age Concern England, London.

Chapter 5

Diabetes mellitus and the Indo-Asians

Introduction

The world is currently experiencing a diabetes mellitus epidemic. During the last 30 years the prevalence of diabetes has tripled. It is estimated that currently 120–140 million people worldwide suffer from it and the number is expected to increase to 300 million, a 2.5 times increase, by 2025. Asia will have the maximum increase in terms of numbers of patients and will also bear the impact of the burden of the disease. Type 2 diabetes accounts for 90–95% of all cases.

In the UK, around 200 000 people have Type 1 diabetes and more than 1 million have Type 2 diabetes. This represents about 3% of the population.

Diabetes and Indo-Asians

There is a worldwide increase in the prevalence of Type 2 diabetes in Indo-Asians. In the UK diabetes is more common among the Indo-Asians compared with the Caucasian population. It is estimated that 17.9% of Indo-Asians aged 24–74 have the disorder while a further 18.7% have impaired glucose intolerance.

The Indo-Asians in the UK originate from the Indian subcontinent (India, Pakistan, Bangladesh, Sri Lanka and Nepal), East Africa and the West Indies. There are marked cultural, social, dietary and religious differences between them. For example, the majority of Hindus and Sikhs are vegetarians and non-smokers while immigrants from Pakistan and Bangladesh are predominantly Muslims and non-vegetarians and either smoke or chew tobacco. However, Indo-Asians universally show the trend for Type 2 diabetes which develops 10 years earlier than in the Caucasian population. They also exhibit a higher propensity for renal and cardiovascular complications.

One of the main risk factors for Type 2 diabetes in the Indo-Asian is the insulin resistance syndrome with central obesity, hyperinsulinaemia, high triglycerides and low HDL-cholesterol. They exhibit evidence of insulin resistance at an early age and the association of insulin resistance and obesity may express itself at a lower level of obesity.

Epidemiology

A house-to-house self-reporting survey of patients with known diabetes conducted in 1984 in the Southall district of west London showed that the age-adjusted prevalence in Indo-Asians was 3.8 times higher than the European cohort. Most Indo-Asians in the survey were Punjabis (Sikhs 57%, Hindus 26%

and Muslims 12%) and were born in India (77%), East Africa (12%) and Pakistan (7%).

Another study carried out in East London in 1985 among Bangladeshi Muslims showed that diabetes was three times more common than in Europeans.

Table 5.1 Countries of origin, religion and life style of Indo-Asians

Country of origin	Religion	Dietary preference	Tobacco use
India			
	Hinduism	Vegetarian	Either
	Sikhism	Vegetarian	None
	Islam	Non-vegetarian	Yes
	Christianity	Non-vegetarian	Yes
Pakistan	Islam	Non-vegetarian	Yes
Bangladesh	Islam	Non-vegetarian	Yes
Sri Lanka	Hinduism	Either	Either
	Buddhism	Vegetarian	Either
East Africa	Hinduism	Vegetarian	None
West Indies	Hinduism	Either	Either

An observational study was carried out on a group of 49 elders (31 women) from the Punjab living in Hertfordshire. The aim of the study was to look into their health and social status. One man and four women (10%) were known to have Type 2 diabetes. Glycosuria was discovered in two men who were previously not known to be diabetic.

Pathophysiology

Type 2 diabetes is a chronic progressive disorder of metabolism characterised by defects of insulin secretion and utilisation. In Type 2 diabetes there is increased concentration of circulating insulin and inadequate pancreatic beta-cell response to hyperinsulinaemia, ultimately leading to beta-cell failure. This leads to increased basal hepatic glucose output and markedly reduced muscle glucose uptake.

Syndrome X (Insulin resistance syndrome)

It has long been recognised that cardiovascular risk factors, which include Type 2 diabetes, hypertension, dyslipidaemia and central obesity can co-exist in the same patient. Reaven (1988) proposed in his Banting lecture that these features were related to hyperinsulaemia and postulated the 'Syndrome X' hypothesis (Fig. 5.1)

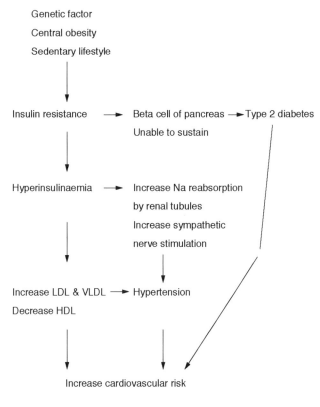

Figure 5.1 Syndrome X

Foetal malnutrition

Nutrition during foetal life and early infancy may be a crucial factor in the development of Type 2 diabetes in later life. The pancreatic beta-cell mass in humans increases more than 130-fold between the 12th week of gestation and the fifth post-natal month, suggesting that the peak beta-cell mass is determined during pregnancy. Nutrition, both maternal and foetal, is the main contributing factor in the growth of the beta-cell mass. Maternal hyperglycaemia, particularly in late pregnancy, leads to neonatal beta-cell hyperplasia while malnutrition, particularly in rats, causes permanent reduction of the beta-cell mass. Fewer beta-cells are also found in human infants of low birth weight which could be a sign of intrauterine malnutrition.

Infantile malnutrition

The combination of malnutrition during foetal life and infancy followed by overnutrition in childhood and adult life predisposes to diabetes in later life. A study carried out in Hertfordshire found that children who were short or thin at birth continued to have low birth weight in their infancy but from seven years onwards had accelerated growth in height and weight. This cohort developed Type 2 diabetes later in life.

A similar study of 500 subjects born in Helsinki between 1924 and 1933 showed that the development of insulin resistance was associated with low birth weight and continued thinness in childhood followed by the development of overweight and Type 2 diabetes in later life.

The thrifty genotype and thrifty phenotype hypothesis

In 1962 Neel first proposed the thrifty genotype hypothesis when the distinction between types 1 and 2 were not defined. He attempted to link the cause of diabetes and obesity with genetic evolutionary development. Neel suggested that the predisposition to obesity could arise from the genetic variations which initially were advantageous in certain environmental conditions like food shortage but later became disadvantageous causing diseases like diabetes. Neel describes this as 'a thrifty genotype rendered detrimental by progress'. It is possible that genetic variation to the predisposition to diabetes mellitus might have been associated with selective advantage at some point in the human evolution. This has been observed among the Pima American Indians of Arizona who have a prevalence of Type 2 diabetes in 60% of their population. Polynesian populations also have a high prevalence of diabetes followed by migrant Indo-Asians.

The thrifty phenotype hypothesis was first proposed by Hales and Barker in 1992. The relationship between foetal and infantile malnutrition and the subsequent development of Type 2 diabetes mellitus is intrinsically linked with maternal malnutrition (Fig 5.2). The high incidence of diabetes in the present generation of middle-aged Indo-Asians could be partly explained by this hypothesis. The parents, particularly the mothers, of this present generation suffered from extreme poverty and malnutrition caused by drought and famine (the Bengal famine of 1943 and the food shortage during World War II). Mass migration and the subsequent race riots of Hindus and Muslims caused by the partition of British India in 1947 did not help matters for several subsequent years. During this period there was mass unemployment and very poor food production in the otherwise fertile planes of the rivers Indus and Ganges.

It can be postulated that the children born in and around this period were severely malnourished. As mentioned before, this could have led to poor development of pancreatic beta cell mass and subsequent insulin undersecretion due to intrauterine programming of the pancreas. Foetal malnutrition triggers the mechanism of nutritional thrift leading to differential growth of different organs with the selective protection of the brain growth. This altered growth pattern has a permanent effect on the structure and function of the body in later life aggravated by increased food consumption and decreased energy spending. The result is obesity, particularly around the trunk, which directly contributes to insulin resistance and the development of Type 2 diabetes mellitus (Fig. 5.3).

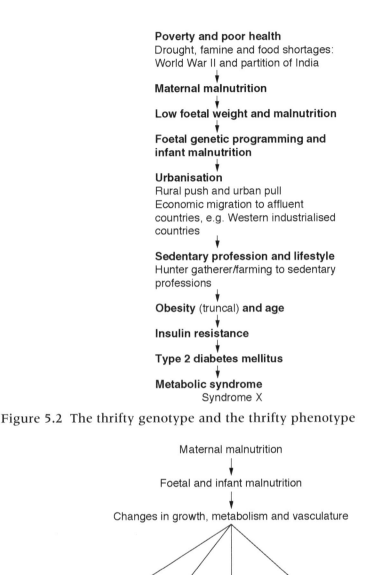

Figure 5.2 The thrifty genotype and the thrifty phenotype

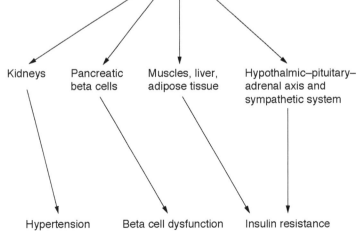

Figure 5.3 Metabolic syndrome X

Complications

There are three studies which have looked into the ethnic and geographical variability of diabetic complications (Table 5.2 and Table 5.3).

Table 5.2 Diabetic complications studies: numbers of subjects

Studies	Indo-Asians	White Europeans
WHO Study (*Diabetologica* 1985)	555	497
Southall Study (*BMJ* 1985)	491	401
Leicester Study (*Diabetic Research & Clinical Practice* 1999)	456	451

Table 5.3 Prevalence rates of diabetic complications among Indo-Asians and whites

	WHO study		Southall study		Leicester study	
	Indians	Whites	Indians	Whites	Indians	Whites
MI	48(9%)	35(7%)	26(7%)	31(7%)	68(15%)	58(13%)
Angina	96(17%)	82(16%)	29(5.7%)	25(5%)	64(14%)	56(12%)
Retinopathy	101(20%)	219(47%)	58(16%)	72(17%)	53(12%)	146(32%)
Cataracts	–	–	58(16%)	72(16%)	45(10%)	23(5%)
PVD	8(1%)	15(5%)	55(16%)	115(29%)	17(4%)	42(9%)
Hypertension	165(30%)	128(26%)	112(29%)	140(29%)	86(18.5%)	85(19.5%)
Renal	37(7%)	47(9%)	–	–	92(20%)	57(13%)

MI = Myocardial infarction; PVD = peripheral vascular disease.

Macrovascular disease

Coronary heart disease (CHD)

The prevalence of myocardial infarction was similar among the Indo-Asian diabetic group and the white European diabetic group in the Southall and Leicester studies. Indo-Asians with diabetes had slightly higher prevalence than the European men and had a 3.3 times greater risk of having a myocardial infarction than their non-diabetic counterparts. The corresponding risk for Europeans was 1.3. Indo-Asians on insulin carried a 9.9 times higher risk than non-diabetic Asians.

Peripheral vascular disease (PVD)

The prevalence of PVD in the Leicester study was low among Indo-Asians (men 3.9%, women 3.5%) when compared with white subjects with diabetes (men 11.5%, women 5.9%). Gangrene and amputation were also found to be lower in the Indo-Asian group (men 1.5%, women 2.4%) compared with white Europeans with diabetes (men 5.7%, women 3.2%). Furthermore, amputation among the Indo-Asian diabetics was confined to the toes, suggesting that the arterial occlusions were more distal. The relative risk for Indo-Asians developing PVD was 0.51.

Cerebrovascular disease (CVD)

The prevalence of CVD in the Leicester study was found to be less among Indo-Asians (men 2.8%, women 1.2%) when compared with white Europeans (men 4.1%, women 2.7%). The adjusted relative risk of Indo-Asians developing CVD was 0.61. For stroke lasting more than 24 hours, the adjusted relative risk was 0.48.

Microvascular disease

Retinopathy

The prevalence of retinopathy in the three studies was lower among the Indo-Asians. In the Leicester Study the prevalence rates for eye disease among the Indo-Asians were 12% (men 10.5%, women 13.3%) while among the white Europeans the rate was 32% (men 31.6%, women 33.5%). The adjusted relative risk for Indo-Asians developing eye disease was 0.31. The prevalence rate for developing cataract, though, was higher among the Indo-Asians (men 10.6%, women 6.4%) when compared with white Europeans (men 6.4%, women 3.2%).

The WHO Study also showed lower prevalence rates of retinopathy among Indo-Asians (20%) when compared with the European group (47%). In contrast, the prevalence rates for retinopathy in the Southall Study were similar in the Indo-Asians (16%) and the Europeans (17%).

Nephropathy

The prevalence rates for renal complications among the Indo-Asians were higher in the Leicester Study. Nephropathy was found in 20% of Indo-Asian subjects (men 24.4%, women 19.1%) compared with 13% of Europeans (men 13.2%, women 11.9%). The prevalence of proteinuria was greater in the Indo-Asian group. The age-adjusted relative risk of developing renal disease was 3.36. The high incidence of end-stage renal disease in the Indo-Asian group will put greater pressure on the renal transplantation service.

Attitude of Indo-Asians towards diabetes and barriers to change

Diet and cultural needs

In this population group, obesity is a sign of prosperity and affluence. It also indicates that the person is not suffering from debilitating illnesses like tuberculosis. Therefore being obese, in the eyes of family and friends, equates with being 'healthy'.

Fasting and feasting are religious needs in both the Muslim and Hindu communities. Muslims fast during the month of Ramadan and can ingest large amounts of high-fat foods and refined carbohydrate when they break their fast. Fasting during Ramadan is relatively safe for diabetic patients on diet and oral hypoglycaemics. They are exempt from fasting but most patients ignore this and fast for their spiritual fulfilment (see below).

A large proportion of daily energy intake among Indo-Asians comes from saturated fats and refined carbohydrate. During feasting, social and emotional pressures are imposed by family and friends to consume large quantities of dairy products such as sweets made from condensed milk, cottage cheese, nuts, ghee and yoghurt.

Smoking and lifestyle

Smoking is common among immigrant men from Pakistan and Bangladesh. Smoking is prohibited during the festival of Ramadan. Smoking cessation schemes should therefore be targeted at Muslim men during this period.

A sedentary lifestyle is popular among the Indo-Asian community and negative attitudes toward exercising are prevalent among first-generation immigrants. Cold and wet British weather and women venturing outdoors without a chaperone are just some of the excuses used against outdoor activities.

Compliance with therapy and follow-up

Traditional (Ayurvedic, Unnani and herbal) and alternative remedies are popular for controlling diabetes among Indo-Asians. Tropical vegetables like bitter gourd (*karela*), 'tindora' and fenugreek (*methi*) seeds have mild hypogly-caemic properties and hence are tried first by the majority of patients. These vegetables have been shown to reduce blood glucose if consumed in large quantity with diabetic medications. A survey carried out in west London showed that 80% of Indo-Asians patients with diabetes attending an outpatient clinic had used some type of alternative therapy for their diabetic management in the previous year.

Using insulin has a cultural stigma and is resisted with vigour. Loss of regular follow-up is common and an important management issue. Patients go 'home' to the Indian subcontinent for prolonged periods and diabetic control during these long holiday breaks is difficult to maintain.

Impact of religious beliefs on diabetic control

Diabetic care and Islam

There are 1.5 million Muslims in the UK and 20% suffer from diabetes. The majority of the Muslim population originates from Pakistan and Bangladesh. During the month of Ramadan (also known as *Ramzan* in the Indian subcontinent), Muslims will fast from dawn to sunset. A pre-dawn meal (*suhr*) and a large meal after sunset are taken. The Muslim calendar follows the lunar cycle of 12 months (354 days). Ramadan falls in the ninth month of the calendar and rotates throughout the seasons. Therefore if Ramadan falls during the winter months the fast will last for 10 hours whereas in the summer it will last for 19 hours. This will have a big impact on diabetic control.

Exemptions from fasting

It is an obligatory requirement for every healthy Muslim to fast. Abstinence from food, drink, smoking and chewing tobacco, oral, aural, nasal medications and intravenous fluids and drugs is practised. However, some individuals are exempt from fasting:

- pre-pubertal children
- the old and infirm
- acutely unwell patients
- those with chronic illnesses for whom fasting may harm their health, e.g. diabetics
- those travelling more than 50 miles in a single journey
- pregnant, nursing and menstruating women
- those with learning difficulties who are unable to understand the purpose of the fast.

Diabetic patients who are advised not to fast include those:

- with 'brittle' Type 1 diabetes
- with concurrent serious pre-morbid conditions like IHD/angina, heart failure, intercurrent infections, etc.
- with history of recurrent diabetic ketoacidosis
- with renal impairment of any severity with risk of dehydration
- who have poor glycaemic control in both Type 1 and Type 2 diabetes
- who are known to be non-compliant with diet and medication.

Prescribing oral hypoglycaemic agents during Ramadan

- Short-acting sulphonylurea (± metformin) should be prescribed and the pre-Ramadan dose should be reversed and taken at the pre-dawn meal and the sunset meal.
- Long-acting sulphonylureas, such as chlorpropamide and glibenclamide, such as should be avoided.

Prescribing insulin during Ramadan

Short-acting insulin should be given before the pre-dawn meal. A combination of short-acting and intermediate-acting insulin should be used before the sunset meal. A drastic reduction of the total amount of insulin is not recommended.

Muslim festivals

- *Eid ul Fitter* follows the end of Ramadan and is the main religious festival. Traditionally the festivities continue for three days and revolve around food, with many dishes having a large sugar content.

- *Eid ul Izha* is the second major Muslim festival and occurs 70 days after *Eid ul Fitter*. Festivities include food with high animal protein content.

Diabetic care and the Hindus

Diabetes was described in Hindu scriptures and Ayurvedic literature several centuries before the birth of Christ. Ancient Hindu physicians had noted that the diabetic patient's urine attracted ants (*medh meah*, translated as 'honeyed urine'). Ayurvedic literature recommends dietary control, herbal remedies and bitter vegetables like *karela* and fenugreek.

Hindu festivals

Hindus have many festivals with fasting and feasting. There is a popular saying that Hindus have 13 festivals in the 12 months of their lunar calendar. The start of the new Hindu calendar may vary. For example, the Hindu Bengali New Year starts in April while the *Devnagri* calendar starts its new year on *Diwali* (festival of lights), which is in November.

Other main festivals include:

- *Navratri* or *Dussehra* in October.
- *Holi* in March/April.
- *Jamnastami* which celebrates Lord Krishna's birthday.
- *Ram-nawmi* which celebrates Lord Rama's birthday.
- *Sivratri* which worships Lord Shiva.

The diabetic team needs to be aware of these major festivals. Patients attending diabetic clinics will not arrive on these festival days.

During all festivals, standard advice on diabetic control should be given.

Diabetic care and the Sikhs

There are 20 million Sikhs worldwide. The word 'Sikh' means disciple of God and they follow the teaching of their 10 gurus. Sikhs believe in one God. Their spiritual head is their religious scripture, the *Sri Guru Granth Sahib*.

Sikh festivals

The Nankshahi calendar starts with the birth of Guru Nanak (1469 AD) who is one of the 10 Sikh gurus.

- *Baisakhi* falls in mid-April to celebrate the start of the Khalsa order.
- *Diwali*, the Hindu festival of lights, is also celebrated by the Sikhs.
- *Maghi* occurs around mid-January.
- *Hola Mohalla*, a mock battle ceremony the day after the Hindu festival of *Holi*.
- *Gurpurbs*, anniversaries of the gurus. Celebration of Guru Nanak's birthday is in November.
- *Akhand Path*, non-stop cover-to-cover reading of the *Sri Guru Granth Sahib*.

Sweets, sugared water or milk, *karah prashad* (sacred pudding) and consecrated food are distributed on these occasions.

The Sikh diet is similar to other Indo-Asian diets in its liberal use of clarified butter (*ghee*). Sikhs do not believe in fasting and there are no religious restrictions on consuming meat. But Sikhism rejects killing of animals as sacrifice or by any means other than a swift death, therefore *halal* or *kosher* meat is forbidden. Many elders in the community are vegetarian.

Alcohol consumption, particularly spirits, can be high among Sikh men and can cause high rates of alcohol-related liver and psychiatric problems. Sikhs do not smoke or chew tobacco.

During festivals, Sikhs should be advised to follow standard dietary and glycaemic advice.

Management

- *Initial screening*: BMI, blood pressure, physical examination, sensory testing, retinal photography and fundoscopy, microalbuminuria
- *Risk factor management*: smoking cessation, hypertension management, dyslipidaemia management
- *Lifestyle management*: diet and calorie restriction, weight reduction, exercise, tobacco consumption, alcohol intake
- *Medical management*: oral antidiabetic therapy, insulin
- *Follow-up*: yearly follow-up, physical examination, Hba1c, microalbuminuria, retinal photography, risk factor management
- *Complication management*: retinopathy, nephropathy, neuropathy
- *Multidisciplinary team management*: diabetologist (hospital consultant and general practice), diabetic nurse, district nurse, dietician, podiatrist, optician, ophthalmologist, vascular surgeon
- *Driving and DVLA.*

Initial screening

The diagnosis of diabetes mellitus should be confirmed by using the WHO criteria and/or glucose tolerance test (Box 5.1). The patient should then be examined and counselled by a diabetic nurse specialist or a diabetologist (GP or hospital consultant).

Box 5.1 Diagnostic criteria for diabetes mellitus (75 g oral glucose tolerance test)

Fasting plasma	<6.1	Normal
Glucose (mmol/L)	>6.1–<7.0	Impaired fasting glucose (IFG)
	>7.0	Diabetes
2-hour plasma	<7.8	Normal
Glucose (mmol/L)	>7.8–11.1	Impaired glucose tolerance (IGT)
	>11.1	Diabetes

Any history of weight loss, polyuria, polydipsia, visual problems, thrush, cardiovascular symptoms, etc., should be sought. Physical examination should include weighing the patient, cardiovascular assessment (including blood pressure), examination of the feet (including sensory testing and pedal pulses). Fundoscopy to elicit retinal changes must be done. Retinal photography must be carried out to record changes in the fundus. Urine testing for glucose and albumin should be carried out. For newly diagnosed diabetics, baseline tests for microalbuminuria should be organised.

Risk factor management

Body mass index is a good indicator of a patient's pre-morbid lifestyle. Obese patients will need counselling from a dietician and a diabetic nurse.

The Joint British Societies Coronary Risk Prediction Chart uses systolic blood pressure, serum total cholesterol to HDL cholesterol ratio and smoking in diabetics for either sex and gives estimation for coronary heart disease (CHD) risk for individuals who have not developed CHD or other major atherosclerotic disease.

Blood pressure should be brought below 140/80 mmHg (British Hypertension Society guidelines) using ACE inhibitors as first-line therapy. Where there is microalbuminuria, blood pressure should be below 125/75 mmHg and treatment should include aspirin, a statin and an ACE inhibitor.

In the UK Prospective Diabetes Study (UK PDS 1998), patients suffering from Type 2 diabetes with a mean age of 56 years were given either a beta-blocker (atenolol) or an ACE inhibitor (captopril) to achieve 'tight' blood pressure control (mean 144/82 mmHg). Treatment was given for 8.4 years. When compared with control (mean 154/87 mmHg), there was significant reduction in diabetic-related death by 32%, stroke by 44%, heart failure by 56% and progression of retinopathy by 37%. The clinical benefit of reducing BP by 10/5 mmHg was greater than that of glycaemic control.

Lifestyle management

Diet and calorie intake

Approximately 80% of Type 2 diabetics are overweight. The association between obesity, complications of diabetes and mortality is well recognised. Calorie restriction and dietary counselling lead to rapid improvement of glycaemic control within 7–10 days. In the UK PDS study (1998), following dietary counselling for three months overweight patients decreased their weight by 7% (from 130% to 123%).

The British Diabetic Association has produced several simple guides for the Indo-Asian population and further details are available from: BDA, 10 Queen Anne Street, London W1M 0BD.

Principles of diabetic diet

- Eat regular meals, including a starchy food like bread, potatoes and cereals.
- Avoid sugar and foods and drinks rich in very refined sugar, such as sweetmeats (*jalebi, burfi*), jaggary, chocolates, etc.

- Eat less fat and avoid deep-fried snacks like samosas, Bombay Mix, pakoras, etc. (Table 5.4)
- Eat more high-fibre food (Table 5.5).
- Take five portions of fruit and vegetables daily.
- Reduce salt intake.
- Drink alcohol in moderation (three units/day for men and two units/day for women). One unit equals half a pint of lager or beer, one pub measure of spirit, e.g. whisky, gin, vodka, sherry, one standard glass of wine.
- Avoid special 'diabetic' products.

Table 5.4 Examples of fat contents and calories

Type	Portions(g)	Fat (g)	Calories (kcal)
Chapatis made without fat	50	1	200
Chapatis made with fat	50	13	330
Lamb curry	170	57	640
Lentil curry (dhal)	170	6	140

Table 5.5 Examples of carbohydrate content

Type	Handy measure	Carbohydrate (g)
Chapati – thick	7–8" diameter	40–45
Chapati – medium	6" diameter	25
Pitta bread	Half	20
Basmati rice	9 tbsp	30
Chick pea curry	7 tbsp	20
Mung dhal	5 tbsp	15
Mixed salad	Small portion	neg
Natural yoghurt	Small portion	10
Mango	1 medium	30

Body mass index (BMI)

BMI is used to grade degrees of obesity and is calculated by dividing weight in kilograms by metres squared (kg/m^2) (Table 5.6).

Table 5.6 Degrees of obesity

BMI grade	BMI range	Degree of obesity
Grade 0	20–24.9	Healthy
Grade I	25–29.9	overweight
Grade II	30–39	clinically obese
Grade III	>40	morbidly obese

Grade 0 is 'desirable' while grade III is severe morbid obesity. Grade I obesity should be treated if the following conditions are present:

- adults under 50 years of age
- diabetes
- truncal or central obesity
- hyperlipidaemia
- hypertension.

Sometimes measurement of a patient's height can be difficult so instead demi-span measurement could be used. The measurement (in centimetres) is taken from the sternal notch to the finger root between the middle and ring fingers while the patient is sitting. The conversion of demispan (cm) to height (m) is done using a conversion chart.

Drugs like orlistat and sibutramine, and gastrointestinal surgical procedures such as Roux-en-Y, are rarely needed.

Tobacco consumption

Tobacco chewing and smoking should be actively discouraged. Oropharyngeal cancers are linked with tobacco chewing and ingestion. Smokers should have access to a smoking cessation clinic for behavioural therapy. Muslim patients should be encouraged to use the fasting month of Ramadan to give up smoking.

Alcohol intake

Alcohol consumption within normal guidelines can be safe for most diabetics. The potential benefit of moderate alcohol consumption (14–21 units per week) in reducing CHD is well known by the public. The effect of alcohol on glycaemic control, weight control and interaction with concurrent medications must be highlighted. 'Low-alcohol' beers, lager and wine are rich in sugars while 'low-sugar' products contain more alcohol and can derange glycaemic control.

Medical management

Oral antidiabetic drugs

Oral antidiabetic drugs are indicated in Type 2 diabetes only if the patient fails to respond adequately to calorie restriction, reduction in carbohydrate intake and increased physical activity for at least three months. Antidiabetic drugs are not a replacement for these lifestyle changes (Tables 5.7 and 5.8).

Table 5.7 Insulin secretagogues

	Dose (daily)	Half-life (h)
Sulphonylureas		
Tolbutamide	0.5–2 g	6–12
Gliclazide	40–320 mg	6–12
Glimepride	1–4 mg	24
Glipizide	2.5–20 mg	12–18
Gliquidone	15–60 mg	6–12
Glibenclamide	5–15 mg	12–24
Chlorpropamide	250–500 mg	>48
Metiglinide analogues		
Nateglinide	60–180 mg tds	2–4
Repaglinide	500 mcg–16 mg	Long acting

Table 5.8 Insulin sensitisers

	Dose	Half-life
Biguanides		
Metformin	500 mg–3 g daily	Short acting
Thiazolidinediones		
Pioglitazone	15–30 mg daily	Long acting
Rosiglitazone	4–8 mg daily	Long acting with metformin
Delayed carbohydrate absorption		
Acarbose	Up to 50 mg tds	Short acting
Guar gum	5 g tds	

The diabetic nurse specialists work closely with the diabetologists both in the hospital and general practice settings and are very useful links for the patients. The new GP contract has been introduced recently in the UK. A very specific protocol to manage diabetic patients has to be followed.

Insulin therapy

Patients who do not achieve ideal control on dietary regimen and maximum antidiabetic medications, may have insulin added to oral therapy or substituted for the oral therapy (Box 5.2). Isophane insulin is usually given at bedtime. Weight gain and hypoglycaemia are the usual complications of insulin therapy (Table 5.9).

Box 5.2 Types of insulin

Highly purified animal insulin – porcine, bovine
Human sequence insulin
Recombinant human insulin analogues

When prescribing highly purified animal insulin, the prescriber should consider the religious needs and cultural values of the patient. Muslim patients should not be prescribed porcine insulin while Hindu patients should not be given either porcine or bovine insulin without their approval and agreement.

Table 5.9 Pharmacokinetics of human insulin preparations

Insulin type	Onset of action	Peak action	Duration of action
Short-acting analogues (Lispro, Aspart)	10–15 minutes	1–2 hours	4–5 hours
Regular	15–30 minutes	2–4 hours	5–8 hours
NPH	1–3 hours	4–6 hours	8–16 hours
Lente	2–3 hours	7–12 hours	12–18 hours
Ultralente	3–4 hours	8–10 hours	12–24 hours
Long-acting analogues (glargine)	1–4 hours	8–12 hours	24 hours
Pre-mixed, 25/75,30/70	15–30 minutes	4–6 hours	8–16 hours
Pre-mixed short-acting analogues, 25/75, 30/70	10–15 minutes	4–6 hours	8–16 hours

Follow-up

Follow-up of Indo-Asian patients can be difficult. Interpreters are available in hospitals but difficult to organise in the community. Family members usually accompany the patients. Leaflets, audio and video cassettes are available in many ethnic languages. Dietary advice regarding ethnic diets is difficult to come by. Dieticians from the ethnic community are few and far between but, when available, they are extremely useful.

When diabetic control is stabilised the patient should have yearly checks on:

- physical examination including blood pressure and BMI
- target organ testing: retina, feet, sensory nerves, pedal pulses
- Hba1c
- microalbuminuria
- retinal photography
- lifestyle management: tobacco smoking or chewing cessation, exercise.

These are specified in the GP contract.

Losing patients to follow-up is not uncommon, particularly when they go 'home' to the Indian subcontinent for prolonged periods. Diabetic control during these visits is less than optimal. Negotiating with the patients on a suitable method of diabetic control and reporting back to the clinic on their return from holiday is crucial.

Multidisciplinary team management

A multidisciplinary team of experts should carry out management of diabetic patients. The diabetic nurse is the co-ordinator of care provision. The team includes the following members.

Core team

- diabetologist (hospital consultant or general practitioner)
- diabetic nurse
- district nurse
- dietician
- podiatrist
- ophthalmologist.

Other members

- vascular surgeon
- nephrologist
- social worker.

Diabetes, driving and the DVLA

The Secretary of State for Transport has responsibility to ensure that all driving licence holders are fit to drive. This responsibility is carried out by the medical advisers at the Drivers Medical Unit of the Driver and Vehicle Licensing Agency (DVLA). The legal basis of fitness to drive is dealt with in the Road Traffic Act 1988 and the Motor Vehicle (Driving Licences) Regulations 1996. Section 92 of the Road Traffic Act 1988 deals with the 'prescribed, relevant and prospective disabilities'. An example of prescribed disability would be epilepsy, relevant disability would be visual field defect while prospective disability would be insulin-dependent diabetes. It is the duty of the licence holder to notify the DVLA of any medical conditions which may affect safe driving. For further information please consult the DVLA website.

Further reading

Chowdhury TA, Grace C and Kopelman G (2003) Preventing diabetes in South Asians (editorial). *BMJ.* **327**: 1059–60.

DVLA (2001) *At a Glance Guide to Current Medical Standards of Fitness to Drive.* DVLA, Swansea.

Ghosh P (1998) South Asian elders – special group with special needs. *Geriatric Med.* **28:** 11–13.

Goenka N, Marwa K, Randava HS, et al. (2001) Diabetic care in the Sikh patient: cultural and clinical aspects. *Br J of Diabetes & Vascular Disease.* **1:** 202–5.

Hale CM, Barker DJP (1991) Fetal and infant growth and impaired glucose tolerance at age 64. *BMJ.* **303:** 1019–22

Hale CN and Barker DJP (2001) The thrifty phenotype hypothesis. *Br Med Bulletin.* **60:** 5–20

Healthy Asian Cooking (1988) *Balance,* the magazine of the British Diabetic Association, London, October.

Mather HM and Keen H (1985) Southall Diabetic Survey; prevalence of known diabetes. *BMJ.* **291:** 1081–4.

Mather HM, Chaturvedi N and Fuller JH (1998) Mortality and morbidity from diabetes in South Asians and Europeans: 11 years follow-up of the Southall Diabetic Survey, London, UK. *Diabetic Med.* **15:** 53–9.

McKeigue PM, Marmaot MG, Syndercombe YD et al. (1988) Diabetes, hyper-insulinaemia and coronary risk factors in Bangladeshis in East London. *Br Heart J.* **660:** 390–6.

Neel JV (1962) Diabetes mellitus: a thrifty genotype rendered detrimental by 'progress'. *Am J Hum Genet.* **14:** 353–62.

Patel N, Drubra U and Chowdhury TA (2002) Special issues in the management of diabetes in South Asians living in the UK. *Modern Diab Mgmt.* **2:** 2–5.

Prantice AM (2003) Intrauterine factors, adiposity, and hyperinsulinaemia (editorial). *BMJ.* **327:** 880–1.

Patel V, Morrissey J, Goenka N et al. (2001) Diabetes care in the Hindu patient: cultural and clinical aspects. *Br J Diabetes & Vascular Disease.* **1:** 132–5.

Roshan M and Burden AC (1993) Diabetic complications and the Indian Asian. *Practical Diabetes.* **10:** 91–3.

Reaven GM (1988) Banting lecture: role of insulin resistance in human disease. *Diabetes.* **37:** 1595–1607.

Riste L, Khan F and Cruickshank K (2001) High prevalence of type 2 diabetes in all ethnic groups, including Europeans, in British inner city. Relative poverty, history, inactivity or 21st century Europe? *Diabetic Care.* **24:** 1377–83.

Samanta A, Burden AC and Jegger C (1999) A comparison of the clinical features and vascular complications of diabetes between migrant Asians and caucasians in Leicester UK. *Diabetic Research and Clinical Practice.* **43:** 167–71.

Shaikh S, James D Morrissey J et al. (2001) Diabetic care and Ramadan: to fast or not to fast? *Br J of Diabetes & VascularDisease,* 2001; **1:** 65–7.

UK Prospective Diabetes Study Group (1998) Efficacy of atenolol and captopril in reducing risk of macro-vascular and micro-vascular complications in Type 2 diabetes. UK PDS 39. *BMJ.* **317:** 713–20.

Whincup PH, Gilg J, Papacosta O et al. (2002) Early evidence of ethnic differences in cardiovascular risk: cross sectional comparison of British South Asian and white children. *BMJ.* **324:**635–8.

Wilke TJ (1993) Early nutrition & diabetic mellitus (editorial). *BMJ.* **306:** 283–4.

World Health Organization Multinational Study of Vascular Disease in Diabetes. Diabetic Drafting Group (1985) Prevalance of small vessel and large vessel disease in diabetic patients from 14 centres. *Diabetologica.* **28:** 615–40.

Chapter 6

Hypertension in Indo-Asians

Introduction

Blood pressure increases with age and accounts for 4.5% of the disease burden around the globe. The prevalence of hypertension increases to over 50% in people aged over 65 years living in the developed world. In this population the high prevalence of diabetes, obesity and dyslipidaemia makes older patients a particularly high-risk group. While hypertension remains the single most modifiable risk factor for cardiovascular disease, regrettably, underdiagnosis, inadequate treatment and poor blood pressure control are also common in the UK. The recent British Hypertension Society guidelines for hypertension give a broad overview of the management of hypertension and emphasise that treatment should include assessment of all cardiovascular risks.

Hypertension in the elderly

For decades there has been considerable controversy about the management of hypertension in older people. Increased mortality secondary to side effects such as postural hypotension has been the primary concern for many physicians. Uncertainty about the benefits of lowering blood pressure in older patients prevented others from treating hypertension in old age.

Over the past few years irrefutable evidence has been published supporting the treatment of hypertension in older patients. The danger of an adverse outcome caused by raised blood pressure is higher in older people compared with younger patients. The benefits of treating hypertension include reductions in mortality and morbidity from cardiovascular and renal disease which outweighs any adverse effects of antihypertensive medications. While there is strong evidence for treating hypertension in people over 60 years of age, the evidence is sparse for patients aged over 80 years.

The management of hypertension requires a holistic approach to cardiovascular risk factors. The relative risk reduction by treating hypertension is around 20% for coronary events and approximately 40% for strokes. Though the awareness of the benefit of treating hypertension in older people has increased, there is still reluctance to treat mild hypertension. There is evidence to support the fact that many elderly patients diagnosed with hypertension do not continue with treatment and those treated are often poorly controlled.

The 24-hour blood pressure control is of the utmost importance in reducing cardiovascular risk. Morning awakening is accompanied with increase in systolic and diastolic blood pressure. There is also a circadian rhythm for cardiovascular risk with a morning peak for ischaemic stroke, myocardial infarction and sudden death. The physiological night-time dip in blood pressure is an important prognostic factor. A dip of less than 10% of the daytime blood pressure is associated with a poor prognosis. Many elderly patients do not exhibit the nocturnal dip. These facts highlight the importance of 24-hour ambulatory blood pressure monitoring rather than the random blood pressure readings used for many patients. There are implications for therapy in the light of these findings with the emphasis on reducing the post-awakening blood pressure when patients are most at risk. The advice to the patient should be to take anti-hypertensive medications on waking rather than after breakfast.

Definition of hypertension

The World Health Organization guidelines define hypertension as a blood pressure >140 mmHg and/or a diastolic blood pressure of >90 mmHg.

Types of hypertension

In elderly patients several types of hypertension are recorded. The various subtypes include sustained systolic hypertension, diastolic hypertension, systolic plus diastolic hypertension and isolated systolic hypertension. As the population ages, newer subtypes are emerging, including white coat hypertension, nocturnal hypertension and pseudo-hypertension.

Essential hypertension

In some patients with hypertension, systolic and diastolic blood pressure rise together. In the absence of any secondary cause, this is defined as essential hypertension. This is the most common variety of hypertension up to the fifth decade and gradually decreases with age. Sustained systolic and diastolic hypertension is more often observed in women.

Isolated systolic hypertension

As arteriosclerosis sets in, there is a relative drop in diastolic blood pressure due to reduced arterial compliance. With age, the elastic fibres and collagen in the larger arteries are replaced by fibrous tissue. This leads to reduced compliance in these vessels, resulting in raised systolic blood pressure. This cascade of events leads to an increase in systolic blood pressure without an increase in diastolic blood pressure. This pattern is called isolated systolic hypertension, defined as sustained systolic blood pressure of >160 mmHg and diastolic blood pressure of <90–95 mmHg.

Diastolic hypertension

Diastolic hypertension is more common in men but decreases with age. It may account for up to 14% of hypertension in the elderly.

White coat hypertension

White coat hypertension is a phenomenon in which blood pressure readings are abnormal when a doctor takes the blood pressure but are lower when taken in the community or by a nurse. This is not a benign phenomenon and merits close supervision of the patient. Ambulatory 24-hour blood pressure monitoring is useful in this group.

Nocturnal hypertension

There is an association of nocturnal blood pressure levels with end-organ damage. The absence of a nocturnal dip in blood pressure below the daytime blood pressure level may be an important risk factor in patients with hypertension.

Pseudo-hypertension

Pseudo-hypertension is rarely seen in elderly patients as, because of heavy calcification, the brachial artery cannot be compressed. It should be suspected where very high blood pressure readings are recorded without much clinical evidence for sustained hypertension.

Hypertension in Indo-Asians

Studies conducted in urban India in the 1950s showed a low prevalence of hypertension of 2–3%. Over the past 50 years the prevalence of hypertension has increased in both rural and urban India. This is, however, not a universal phenomenon as some rural communities in developing countries do not express the same trend of increase in blood pressure with age.

More recent studies have shown a higher figur, with prevalence ranging from 26% in Southern Pakistan to 31% in South India. Changes in lifestyle and affluence have led to an increase in the prevalence of hypertension in the Indo-Asian population. This increase is most pronounced in Indo-Asians who emigrated to developed countries.

In the UK hypertension is twice as common in Indo-Asians as in the Caucasian population. The reason for this increase is not clear. Genetic differences, effects of migration, change in environment and dietary changes may have some bearing along with the confounding effect of social class.

Undetected hypertension is more common in Indo-Asians. It is noticeable that communities with a higher prevalence of hypertension are less likely to have it detected and managed. Several factors including social, economic and cultural influences could be responsible for this observation.

There are differences within the ethnic groups from the Indian subcontinent, reflecting multiple influences including genetic predisposition. Sikhs are more predisposed to hypertension compared with Hindus, with Muslims being similar to the Caucasian population. Overall, Indian men have higher diastolic blood pressure than the general population but men of Bangladeshi and Pakistani origin have lower mean systolic blood pressure. Some of these differences may be exaggerated by the fact that some ethnic groups have a relatively younger population. Pakistani females tend to have higher blood pressure than the general population whereas Bangladeshi women have lower mean systolic blood pressure.

Risk factors may also vary between the ethnic groups, as smoking is common in Muslims and is not a risk factor in Sikhs who are forbidden to smoke by their religion. Muslims, on the other hand, are prohibited from consuming alcohol while Sikhs have a relatively higher consumption of alcohol. The southern Indian population has high numbers of vegetarians, whereas the Punjabi population of Pakistani origin has a high meat intake. Cholesterol levels are highest in Bangladeshi men and lowest in Gujrati Hindus. These differences may have some bearing on hypertension and the expression of its complications. Despite all these differences, all four main groups of Indo-Asians share the tendency to diabetes, central obesity, hyperinsulinaemia and hypertriglyceridaemia.

Obesity and lack of exercise are particularly common in Indo-Asians along with impairment of glucose tolerance. Type 2 diabetes is widespread and its combination with hypertension leads to early complications such as renal failure and coronary heart disease. Ocular and neurological complications such as stroke are also more common, hence the need for tighter control on blood pressure and cardiovascular risk factors.

The insulin resistance syndrome is more common in Indo-Asians. High triglycerides, low HDL-cholesterol ratio, central obesity plus the high prevalence of diabetes make these patients a high-risk group. Indo-Asians are more prone to complications secondary to hypertension, including ischaemic heart disease and stroke. Differences in the composition and stability of atherosclerotic plaques along with other thrombogenic tendencies may be responsible for the high morbidity and mortality from vascular disease. Thus it is plausible that a lower threshold for intervention is required for initiating hypertension treatment in Indo-Asians. Evidence from predominantly Caucasian populations could not be confidently extrapolated to the Indo-Asian population living in the UK. More work is required to answer these questions.

What is normal blood pressure for Indo-Asians?

There seems to be no difference in the definition for hypertension between Indo-Asians and Caucasians. The cut-off for high blood pressure is the same for both groups. However, people over the age of 60 years have higher risks of complications secondary to hypertension. The risk of experiencing a morbid event is twice as high in Indo-Asians as in the Caucasian population.

The prevalence of Type 2 diabetes in Indo-Asians is high and the British Diabetic Association recommends adequate blood pressure control below 140 mmHg systolic and 80 mmHg diastolic. In diabetic patients with nephropathy and microalbuminuria, the cardiovascular risk doubles and the recommendation of the US Joint National Committee on Prevention, Evaluation, and Treatment of High Blood Pressure is 120/75 mmHg. The British Hypertension Society's 2004 guidelines and data from intervention trials in high-risk patients, e.g. with stroke, support a policy of 'the lower, the better'. Ideally, in high-risk patients, the lowest tolerated blood pressure should be the aim.

With a high incidence of diabetes, ischaemic heart disease and dyslipidaemia, several issues need consideration in relation to Indo-Asians. It is plausible that, in Indo-Asians, complications of hypertension may occur at a lower threshold compared with Caucasians. Having a worse prognosis and being more prone to complications, they may need intervention at a lower blood pressure as they would be at high risk. There are no clear data to support or refute this view and more work is needed to look at different thresholds for intervention in relation to the ethnic background of patients. The lower cut-off for treating hypertension in Indo-Asians remains unclear and there are no recommendations in this respect.

Lifestyle measures including weight loss and exercise should be at the heart of all management regimens. Though there is limited data on the benefits of exercise in Indo-Asians, reducing risk factors by exercise is not well described.

There is a wealth of information showing varied responses to antihypertensive treatment based on ethnic differences. Afro-Caribbean patients are more sensitive to salt restriction and more responsive to diuretics and calcium antagonists. There is blunted response to angiotensin-converting enzyme (ACE) inhibitors and beta-blockers in this group. Though the evidence is limited, Indo-Asians seem to respond to antihypertensive treatment in a similar way to the white population.

Target organ damage and ethnic differences

Evidence for end-organ damage is an important aspect of management while treating hypertensive patients, as the risks escalate with the involvement of target organs. The presence of left ventricular hypertrophy is an important risk factor but should ideally be diagnosed on the basis of echocardiography rather than an electrocardiogram. Left ventricular hypertrophy associated with high blood pressure is an independent risk factor for poor prognosis. It is a strong predictor of cardiovascular morbidity and mortality, even more than hypertension itself. It is associated with stroke, myocardial infarction, atherosclerotic vascular disease and cardiac arrhythmias. Presence of left ventricular hypertrophy in an Indo-Asian would increase the risks several-fold, particularly if associated with insulin resistance syndrome. Heart failure, angina and myocardial infarction are other effects on the heart secondary to hypertension. Peripheral vascular disease could be the end result of chronic hypertension.

Other examples of end-organ damage include renal impairment, proteinuria, fundal haemorrhages, papilloedema and retinopathy. Neurological problems secondary to hypertension include cerebrovascular accident, transient ischaemic attack and dementia.

Box 6.1 Issues to bear in mind while treating hypertension in patients from ethnic minorities

---

- Hypertension is common
- Ratio of undetected hypertension is higher than in Caucasians
- Indo-Asians are a high-risk group
- Obesity and lack of exercise are important risk factors
- It is essential to check for impaired glucose tolerance

Diagnosis of hypertension

Hypertension is diagnosed on three measurements over a period, depending upon the readings and risk factors. Blood pressure should be measured in both sitting and standing postures. For treatment decisions, standing blood pressure readings should be the guide for management in older patients. An average of two readings is recommended. A detailed history and a thorough physical examination are recommended for every patient.

The 2004 British Hypertension Society's guidelines give specific targets for normal blood pressure (Table 6.1) and for diagnosis of hypertension (Table 6.2).

Table 6.1 Normal blood pressure levels as recommended by the British Hypertension Society

	Systolic blood pressure (mmHg)	Diastolic blood pressure (mmHg)
Optimal	<120	<80
Normal	<130	<85
High normal	130–139	85–89

Table 6.2 Hypertension and grades of hypertension as recommended by the British Hypertension Society

Grade	Systolic blood pressure (mmHg)	Diastolic blood pressure (mmHg)
Grade 1 or mild	140–159	90–99
Grade 2 or moderate	160–179	100–109
Grade 3 or severe	180 or over	110 or over

In the elderly between the ages of 60 and 75 years with blood pressure <130 mmHg systolic and <85 mmHg diastolic, it is recommended that blood pressure be checked every five years. Those with readings between 130–139 mmHg systolic and 85–89 mmHg diastolic should have their blood pressure remeasured at least annually. All patients with elevated or borderline blood pressure require advice on lifestyle modifications. For borderline cases where drug therapy is not immediately required, annual blood pressure monitoring and cardiovascular risk stratification are recommended. If the systolic pressure is 140–159 mmHg or the diastolic pressure 90–99 mmHg the patient should be offered treatment with antihypertensive drugs provided there are no complications secondary to hypertension or diabetes. With sustained hypertension, i.e. blood pressure of 160/100 mmHg, treatment with antihypertensive medications is recommended. In patients in whom ambulatory readings are taken, mean daytime blood pressure is preferred and this reading is on average 5–10 mmHg lower than the surgery or hospital blood pressures.

In non-diabetic patients, the minimum acceptable level for controlled hypertension is 150/90 mmHg. The goals for blood pressure treatment should be systolic blood pressure of <140 mmHg and diastolic pressure <85 mmHg. However, in patients with diabetes mellitus, treatment is recommended if systolic blood pressure is 140 mmHg and diastolic pressure 90 mmHg or over. If diabetes and renal disease co-exist the recommended optimal blood pressure goals are systolic pressure <130 mmHg and diastolic pressure <80 mmHg.

For people over the age of 75, a blood pressure check should be performed as part of the annual health check. However, for Indo-Asians in the 60–75 age group, general practitioners should develop a strategy for active case finding.

Investigations

Investigations in patients with hypertension need to be organised with a view to excluding a secondary cause and determining other cardiovascular risk factors.

Looking for secondary causes for hypertension is fruitful only in a minority of elderly patients. In some older patients hypertension is secondary to renovascular disease. This should be suspected in patients with co-existing peripheral vascular disease, cerebrovascular disease and/or coronary artery disease. In this group renal artery stenosis can occur and could influence blood pressure control.

Risk assessment depends upon several factors including family history, age, gender, smoking, glucose tolerance, cholesterol/HDL ratio and BMI. Patients with cerebrovascular or cardiovascular disease have a much higher risk of adverse outcome.

A patient's clinical risks as well as associated pathologies would determine the need for investigations. Basic screening in elderly patients with hypertension should include the following:

- full blood count
- urea, serum potassium and serum creatinine
- blood glucose
- total cholesterol/HDL ratio and triglycerides
- twelve-lead electrocardiogram
- chest X-ray
- urinalysis.

Routine echocardiography is only recommended in specific circumstances.

Complications

The risks of cardiovascular complications secondary to hypertension increase with age.

Hypertension is silent in the majority of patients and this could predispose to suboptimal treatment, leading to serious consequences. The main determinants of hypertension-related risks include level of blood pressure, presence of other cardiovascular risk factors, age and target organ damage. Wide pulse pressure has been shown to be a risk marker in elderly patients.

There is sufficient evidence to show the benefits of treating systolic and diastolic blood pressure, one of which is a reduction in cardiovascular complications. The most common cardiovascular complications secondary to hypertension include ischaemic heart disease, heart failure, left ventricular hypertrophy and left ventricular diastolic dysfunction. Ischaemic or haemorrhagic stroke, transient ischaemic attack, dementia, retinopathy, renal failure and peripheral vascular disease are some of the other common complications related to long-standing hypertension. Although antihypertensive treatment reduces the risk for first stroke, information is scarce on the protective effect of antihypertensive treatment on recurrent strokes.

Benefits of treating hypertension in older people

In the Western populations hypertension increases with age and the prevalence is more than 50% in people aged over 65 years. This is in sharp contrast to people living in Third World countries. Treating hypertension is cost-effective in older people. It reduces the risk of heart failure by half and the incidence of stroke and heart attacks. Reduction in stroke is the most important benefit from treating hypertension. In elders of Indo-Asian origin, early detection and treatment of hypertension would be highly desirable.

Many elderly patients with blood pressure of 140/90 mmHg or more would require antihypertensive therapy. The decision to treat does not depend solely on the blood pressure readings. The presence of associated pathology, cardiovascular risks and evidence of end-organ involvement influence the decision to intervene at an early stage. The presence of vascular disease increases the risks and hence these patients are candidates not only for antihypertensive therapy but also antiplatelet and lipid-lowering therapy.

The benefits from intervention are much greater in patients with high risks. A tighter blood pressure control is desirable in high-risk groups, especially in those with Type 2 diabetes, as shown in the UK Prospective Diabetes Study (UK PDS). In some elderly patients this may be difficult to achieve but even a small reduction in blood pressure would be beneficial. A J-shaped relation exists between blood pressure and stroke and hence caution should be exercised in the elderly and especially the very elderly patient.

Lifestyle changes

Lifestyle changes are beneficial in the management of hypertension and may reduce the need for medications. However, in older patients there are several obstacles to achieving this goal. This is particularly the case in patients from Indo-Asian communities.

Language barriers and social pressures can make lifestyle change difficult to implement. Written and verbal instructions may be needed and every effort should be made to ensure that the message has been communicated effectively. Use of interpreters could be invaluable in some patients where language difficulties are encountered. Input from dieticians with experience in Indo-Asian dietary habits is desirable. Increased physical activity and smoking cessation should be part of therapy protocol.

Physical exercise

There is ample evidence to show the cardiovascular benefits of exercise. Increased physical activity has several beneficial effects including reduction of systolic and diastolic blood pressure, reduction in mean serum insulin, BMI and triglyceride levels. To benefit from exercise, 30 minutes of moderate exercise is recommended at least five times per week.

There is a wide variation in physical activity within the Indo-Asian community. The Asian population in the UK has an overall lower level of physical activity than the white population. According to the 1999 census, only 12–19% of Indo-Asian men participate in brisk walking as compared with 28% of the general population. The figure for the Indo-Asian female population is only around 10% as compared with 22% in the general population. Though the data are lacking, anecdotal evidence suggests that there is a substantially lower level of physical activity in elders of Indo-Asians origin as compared with the elderly white population. Interestingly, Asians in India are more physically active than their counterparts in the UK.

Diet and salt consumption

Age-associated increase in blood pressure could be checked by lifestyle modifications including a diet high in fruits, vegetables and whole grains.

Reduction in salt intake of less than 5 g per day can lead to a modest reduction in blood pressure. This effect may be greater in older people due to their greater sensitivity to salt intake. On the other hand, intensive behavioural intervention is less likely to be of benefit in older people. There are no studies that have addressed this issue in relation to Indo-Asians and the long-term benefits of salt restriction remain unclear.

Alcohol

Excessive alcohol intake is an important risk factor for high blood pressure. The increase in blood pressure secondary to alcohol rises with age and can cause resistance to antihypertensive therapy. Alcohol intake varies between the various ethnic groups. Sikhs have a significantly higher consumption of alcohol than Muslims.

Weight reduction

Obesity is a common problem in Indo-Asians and may be more serious in some communities, e.g. people of Punjabi origin. Reduced total fat along with reduction in weight has been shown to be beneficial and is a part of general recommendations. Patients with a BMI of 23 kg/m^2 or over should be actively encouraged to lose weight but it is unrealistic to expect older hypertensive patients to achieve significant weight loss. There is no evidence for the efficacy of weight loss as a treatment modality in older patients.

Stopping smoking

Smoking is a risk factor for cardiovascular disease and in the short term can increase blood pressure. Discontinuation of smoking is an essential part of treating hypertension. There is high incidence of smoking in some Indo-Asian communities. It is a significant problem in Bangladeshi men and Gujrati Hindus but not in the Sikh community. Smoking is uncommon in females of Indo-Asian origin residing in the UK.

Drug therapy

Drug therapy for hypertension is recommended for grade I hypertension (*see* Table 6.2) provided there are no complications secondary to hypertension or diabetes. With sustained hypertension, i.e. blood pressure of 160/100 mmHg, treatment with antihypertensive medications is recommended along with non-pharmacological measures. For most patients a target of <140 mmHg systolic and <85 mmHg diastolic blood pressure is recommended. In patients with diabetes, renal impairment or cardiovascular disease, a lower target of <130/80 mmHg is recommended.

There is greater use of drugs in older patients due to increased co-morbidity. Though medications offer enhanced life expectancy, they may hinder functional independence and quality of life. Elderly patients are at particular risk because of the high incidence of adverse drug reactions and problems with poor drug compliance. These issues may be more important when managing hypertension in Indo-Asians.

There is no evidence that Indo-Asians respond to antihypertensive medications differently from the Caucasian population. The beneficial effects of ACE inhibitors may be more desirable in Indo-Asians with ischaemic heart disease as these drugs have benefits beyond those seen by reduction of blood pressure.

The largest randomised trial of treatment, the Antihypertensive and Lipid-Lowering Treatment to Prevent Heart Attack Trial (ALLHAT), confirms the recommendation that a thiazide diuretic is at least as effective as more expensive medications in older people. The trial suggests that most patients would require two or more drugs to control blood pressure but that control is more difficult in older patients.

Most elderly patients with hypertension will require at least two blood pressure-lowering drugs to reach the desired blood pressure control. As a general rule, combination of drugs in smaller doses may be advantageous as the side effects may be low compared with larger doses of a single agent. The Swedish Trial in Old Patients with Hypertension-2 (STOP-2) showed that blood pressure and end-point reduction could be achieved by combination of diuretic and a beta-blocker or ACE inhibitors or long-acting dihydropyridine calcium antagonists. Many patients will require three antihypertensive drugs to achieve the target blood pressure. One of these should be a diuretic in order to counteract the fluid retention caused by other drugs. Drug therapy depends upon multiple factors, especially associated pathologies.

Table 6.3 shows the British Hypertension Society recommended algorithm for the rationalisation of drug treatment. In this AB/CD algorithm each letter refers to a class of antihypertensive medication.

Table 6.3 British Hypertension Society recommended algorithm for the management of hypertension

AB/CD rule	Class of antihypertensive medicine
A	Angiotensin-converting enzyme inhibitors (ACEI)
B	Beta-blocker
C	Calcium antagonist
D	Diuretic

The white population and people younger than 55 years of age have higher renin compared with older people of the black population. Hence initial therapy with A or B drugs would be more effective. The C or D groups of drugs seem to be better for older people or black people of any age. In uncomplicated patients with poor initial response, the drug could be changed, whereas in complicated patients with poor blood pressure control, the addition of another agent is recommended. If two drugs are required in combination then A or B + C or D would be desirable. For resistant hypertension the combination of A or B + C + D is recommended. If hypertension is still poorly controlled then A + B + C + D and/or the addition of an alpha-blocker or low-dose spironolactone would be desirable.

Ideally, four weeks should be the minimum observation period to determine the effect of a new antihypertensive drug. Long-acting drugs may improve compliance.

Thiazide diuretics

Low-dose thiazide diuretics have been recommended as first-line therapy in older people and this has been reaffirmed by the ALLHAT results. Thiazides have been shown to reduce morbidity and mortality in older patients. Their use in elderly patients has led to reductions in stroke, coronary artery disease and cardiovascular as well as all-cause mortality. They are considerably less expensive than most hypertensive drugs. Hyponatraemia, hypokalaemia, gout and hypocalcaemia are some of the metabolic problems which limit their use. It is recommended that serum potassium and sodium should be measured within 4–6 weeks of commencing thiazide diuretics. Some antihypertensive trials in the elderly have used thiazides in combination with potassium or potassium-sparing diuretics in combination, with favourable results. The use of thiazide diuretics is not recommended in renal failure, especially when serum creatinine is >250 μmol/L, when a loop diuretic is more effective.

In elderly patients with high prevalence of lower urinary tract symptoms, thiazide diuretics may worsen urinary incontinence. This may not be readily acceptable to some Indo-Asian groups such as elderly Muslims. Urinary frequency or incontinence may interfere with their daily ritual of praying five times a day.

Beta-blockers

These drugs help to reduce cerebrovascular events but are less effective in terms of other end-points. In the elderly they are not as effective as thiazide diuretics, as shown by a number of outcome trials. They are less effective in systolic hypertension and as monotherapy in older people and their action may be blunted in smokers.

Beta-blockers are not the first choice of therapy in the elderly as age-related changes blunt the responsiveness of the beta-adrenergic receptors. Beta-blockers are contraindicated in many elderly patients with asthma, chronic obstructive pulmonary disease and peripheral vascular disease. Depression, memory defects and lethargy limit their use in many patients. They can adversely affect the glucose and lipid profiles, an important issue to consider when treating Indo-Asians.

Calcium antagonists

The results of the ALLHAT trial dismiss any concerns about the use of calcium antagonists in the treatment of hypertension. Long-acting dihydropyridine calcium antagonists are well tolerated in the elderly and have efficacy similar to beta-blockers or thiazide diuretics in prevention of cardiovascular events. They are recommended as drugs of choice in patients with isolated systolic hypertension. Short-acting dihydropyridines have been associated with major adverse effects and their use should be avoided. Dihydropyridines and some calcium channel antagonists may worsen heart blocks and adversely affect heart failure.

Angiotensin-converting enzyme inhibitors (ACEI)

Elderly people have lower renin levels and hence abnormalities of the renin-angiotensin system are less likely to be the cause of hypertension. Low renin also explains the reason for the elderly person's susceptibility to sodium load.

ACEI have proven effectiveness in blood pressure reduction. They can reduce cardiovascular mortality and morbidity after myocardial infarction, especially with accompanying left ventricular systolic dysfunction. In the STOP-2 trial ACEI had similar efficacy to thiazide diuretics and beta-blockers. However, the incidence of myocardial infarction and heart failure was significantly less than in patients receiving calcium antagonists.

ACEI have also been proven to be useful in patients with diabetes and they are the drugs of choice in diabetic patients with hypertension. In the Heart Outcomes Prevention Evaluation (HOPE) study, ramipril reduced the incidence of stroke, heart failure and cardiovascular death in high-risk patients. The incidence of myocardial infarction, revascularisation, development of diabetes and diabetic microvascular complications was reduced. More recently, the ACEI perindopril has shown benefits in patients with cerebrovascular disease when used with a thiazide diuretic.

Renal artery stenosis is an uncommon cause of hypertension in the elderly and broadly a contraindication for the use of ACEI. It should be suspected if there is generalised peripheral vascular disease, renal impairment without a cause, unequal renal size on ultrasound, elevation of serum creatinine by ACEI or poorly controlled hypertension. Occasionally these patients present with recurrent pulmonary oedema. In patients with renal artery stenosis, calcium channel blockers and alpha-blockers are the drugs of choice.

ACEI are associated with the risk of worsening renal functions, especially in elderly patients with renovascular disease. Hence serum creatinine should be checked within two weeks of commencing ACEI. In patients with serum creatinine above 150 µmol/L, close monitoring is recommended.

Angiotensin II antagonists

This class of drugs is similar to ACEI with the exception that they do not have cough as a common side effect. Their use is mainly as an alternative therapy to ACEI in patients with cough, angio-oedema or intolerance. Robust evidence for their efficacy in preventing cardiovascular end-points in hypertension is still awaited.

Alpha-blockers

Alpha-blockers are useful in elderly hypertensive patients with prostatism and are effective in reducing blood pressure. The evidence is lacking for their efficacy in preventing cardiovascular end-points. There have been concerns following the results of the ALLHAT trial as a higher proportion of patients developed heart failure while being treated with the alpha-blocker doxazosin. Hence, caution needs to be exercised with their use in elderly hypertensive patients.

Other drugs

In poorly controlled hypertension alternative medications would be needed. These include hydralazine, minoxidil, clonidine and methyldopa.

Aspirin

Aspirin has shown benefit in hypertensive patients. The Hypertension Optimal Treatment (HOT) trial showed benefits of aspirin in hypertensive patients with controlled blood pressure. In this trial 75 mg of aspirin a day in patients aged 50 years and over reduced cardiovascular events by 9% and myocardial infarction by 15%. In the Thrombosis Prevention Trial for primary prevention with aspirin 75 mg a day, there was a 16% reduction in all cardiovascular events and 20% reduction in myocardial infarction but no effect on fatal events. There was a significant risk of bleeding in both trials and this should be carefully considered when treating elderly patients. Hence low-dose aspirin is recommended for secondary prevention of ischaemic heart disease and for primary prevention in patients over 50 years of age.

Statins

Statins are recommended when attempting to reduce cardiovascular risks in patients with accompanying dyslipidaemia. They are recommended for patients with high blood pressure with history of cardiovascular disease, irrespective of baseline total cholesterol or low-density lipoprotein. They are recommended for primary prevention in patients with hypertension where the 10-year risk of cardiovascular disease exceeds 20%. The use of statins for primary prevention in patients aged over 80 years is debatable. Total cholesterol concentration of <5.0 mmol/L or low-density lipoprotein of <3.0 mmol/L is acceptable as the minimum requirement.

Summary

Indo-Asians seem to respond to antihypertensive treatment in the same way as the white population. However, in these patients there is a high incidence of insulin resistance syndrome with high triglycerides, low HDL-cholesterol and central obesity plus high prevalence of diabetes. These issues should be considered when choosing a treatment option. Drugs which improve this metabolic imbalance should be the first choice and include ACEI, angiotensin II receptor antagonists and alpha-blockers.

Drugs which have neutral effect on lipids and glucose metabolism should be the next choice. There is evidence that treatment with diuretics and beta-blockers further increases insulin resistance. This increases the risk of developing Type 2 diabetes or impaired glucose tolerance, both of which are associated with increased risk of coronary heart disease. However, it remains unclear whether diabetes mellitus induced by beta-blockers or thiazide diuretics is associated with increased risk of coronary heart disease.

Many elderly patients are early risers and this is particularly the case with Muslims who get up before sunrise for their morning prayers. These patients should be advised to take their antihypertensive medications on waking rather than waiting for breakfast.

Box 6.2 Special considerations for drug therapy in older people

- More frequent assessment
- Multiple drugs are usually required
- Start at the lowest possible dose
- Slow titration is key to success
- Look out for postural hypotension
- Elderly are more vulnerable to adverse drug reactions
- Poor drug compliance is common

Follow-up

The follow-up for patients with adequately controlled blood pressure depends on several factors. Frailty of the patient, severity of hypertension and the drugs used to control blood pressure generally determine the frequency of follow-up. For patients who are stabilised on treatment, a six-monthly follow-up is recommended when drug compliance and the side effects of medications should be reviewed. Apart from monitoring blood pressure, weight should be checked and advice on lifestyle reinforced. Testing for proteinuria is recommended annually.

Compliance

Long-term compliance with medications is a major cause for concern in the management of hypertensive patients and especially in Indo-Asians. It is estimated that this problem accounts for over 50% of patients who have poor blood pressure control. There are many reasons for non-compliance. In Indo-Asians, lack of understanding of the diagnosis may be the main contributing factor.

Some issues surrounding poor compliance could be improved by counselling, use of compliance aids, using long-acting medications and reducing the number of doses per day and paying particular attention to the side effects. Information leaflets in different languages and the availability of interpreters are of paramount importance.

The very elderly

The case for treating patients up to 80 years of age is fairly clear but evidence is lacking for older patients. The decision to treat hypertension or to withhold medications in very elderly hypertensive patients depends upon individual risk/benefit assessment.

In the SHEP study, treating patients over 80 years of age with isolated systolic hypertension was associated with a 45% reduction in stroke incidence. The Hypertension in the Very Elderly Trial (HYVET) is looking at the benefits of antihypertensive therapy in patients over the age of 80. There are some data to suggest that patients over 80 with hypertension live longer than those with normal blood pressure.

There are no data to guide use of medications in institutionalised frail elderly patients with hypertension. The decision to withdraw or withhold therapy in this cohort depends on several factors including level of frailty, dependence and associated pathologies. Age by itself should not be the only deciding factor and decisions should be made on an individual basis.

Cognitive impairment and hypertension

Hypertension along with other cardiovascular effects is a possible risk factor for cognitive impairment. Early intervention and adequate treatment can reduce this risk. On the other hand, low diastolic blood pressure is associated with dementia.

Hence there are doubts about initiating antihypertensive therapy in very elderly patients with established dementia. There is also controversy over withdrawing antihypertensive therapy in these patients as no clear data from clinical trials are available. Moderate to severe cognitive impairment can also affect the management of hypertension, especially in the form of poor compliance with treatment.

Recommendations

It is proven beyond doubt that there are important differences in prevalence, aetiology, co-morbidity and end-organ damage between the Caucasian and Indo-Asian populations in the UK. These factors, along with hypertension-related mortality and morbidity in the Indo-Asian population, mean that the ethnic origin of patients must be considered before treatment is contemplated.

There is a general lack of information in relation to hypertension in people of Indo-Asian origin. The findings from the European population cannot be extrapolated to the Indo-Asian population. Research is urgently needed to clarify some of the questions that have remained unanswered for decades.

Detection and management of hypertension in the Indo-Asian community are a challenge for healthcare workers and health planners. There are substantial gaps in the detection and management of hypertension which require strategies taking into account the different cultural backgrounds of the target community. The key is to increase awareness in the target communities and their healthcare workers and focus on modifiable vascular risk factors so prevalent in patients of Indo-Asian origin. Advances in living standards and social class, along with better awareness of medical problems, are likely to show improvement in the management of hypertension in Indo-Asians.

Further reading

ALLHAT Collaborative Research Group (2002) Major outcome in high-risk hypertensive patients randomized to angiotensin converting enzyme inhibitors or calcium channel blockers vs diuretics: the Antihypertensive and Lipid Lowering Treatment to prevent Heart Attack Trial (ALLHAT). *JAMA.* **288**: 2981–97.

Amery A, Birkenhäger W, Brixko P et al. (1985) Mortality and morbidity results from the European Working Party on High Blood Pressure in the Elderly trial. *Lancet.* **1**: 1349–54.

Anand SS, Yousaf S, Vuksan V et al. (2000) Difference in risk factors, athero-sclerosis, and cardiovascular disease between ethnic groups in Canada: the study of health assessment and risk in ethnic groups (SHARE). *Lancet.* **356**: 279–84.

Balarajan R (1991) Ethnic differences in mortality from ischaemic heart disease and cerebrovascular disease in England and Wales. *BMJ.* **302**: 560–4.

Barber JH, Beevers DG, Fife R et al. (1979) Blood-pressure screening and supervision in general practice. *BMJ.* **1**: 843–6.

Blacher J, Staessen JA, Girerd X et al. (2000) Pulse pressure not mean pressure determines cardiovascular risk in older hypertensive patients. *Arch Intern Med.* **160**: 1085–9.

Braith RW, Pollock ML, Lowenthal DT, Graves JE and Limacher MC (1994) Moderate- and high-intensity exercise lowers blood pressure in normotensive subjects 60 to 79 years of age. *Am J Cardiol.* **73**: 1124–8.

British Diabetic Association (1998) Joint British recommendations on prevention of coronary heart disease in clinical practice. *Heart.* **80** (suppl 2): S1–S29.

Bulpitt CJ, Fletcher AE, Amery A et al. (1994) The Hypertension in the Very

Elderly Trial (HYVET). Rationale, methodology and comparison with previous trials. *Drugs Ageing.* **5**: 171–83.

Cappuccio FP, Cook DG, Atkinson RW and Strazzullo P (1997) Prevalence, detection and management of cardiovascular risk factors in different ethnic groups in South London. *Heart.* **78**: 555–63.

Cruickshank JK, Jackson SH, Bannan LT, Beevers DG, Beevers M and Osbourne VL (1983) Blood pressure in black, white and Asian factory workers in Birmingham. *Postgrad Med J.* **59**: 622–6.

Curb JD, Pressel SL, Cutler JA et al. (1996) Effect of diuretic-based antihypertensive treatment on cardiovascular disease risk in older diabetic patients with isolated systolic hypertension. Systolic Hypertension in the Elderly Program Cooperative Research Group. *JAMA.* **276**: 1886–92.

Dahlof B, Lindholm LH, Hansson L, Schersten B, Ekbom T and Wester PO (1991) Morbidity and mortality in the Swedish Trial in Old Patients with Hypertension (STOP-Hypertension). *Lancet.* **338**: 1281–5.

Dhawan J and Bray CL (1997) Asian Indians, coronary artery disease, and physical exercise. *Heart.* **78**: 550–4.

Dunder K, Lind L, Zethelius B, Berglund L and Lithell H (2003) Increase in blood glucose concentration during antihypertensive treatment as a predictor of myocardial infarction: population based cohort study. *BMJ.* **326**: 681–4.

Forette F, Seux ML, Staessen JA et al. (1998) Prevention of dementia in randomised double-blind placebo-controlled Systolic Hypertension in Europe (Syst-Eur) trial. *Lancet.* **352**: 1347–51.

Hansson L, Zanchetti A, Carruthers SG et al. (1998) Effects of intensive blood-pressure lowering and low-dose aspirin in patients with hypertension: principal results of the Hypertension Optimal Treatment (HOT) randomised trial. HOT Study Group. *Lancet.* **351**: 1755–62.

Hansson L, Lindholm LH, Ekbom T et al. (1999) Randomised trial of old and new antihypertensive drugs in elderly patients: cardiovascular mortality and morbidity the Swedish Trial in Old Patients with Hypertension-2 study. *Lancet.* **354**: 1751–6.

Heart Outcomes Prevention Evaluation Study Investigators (2000) Effects of an angiotensin-converting-enzyme inhibitor, ramipril, on death from cardiovascular causes, myocardial infarction, and stroke in high-risk patients. *N Engl J Med.* **319**: 630–5.

Hooper L, Bartlett C, Smith GD and Ebrahim S (2000) Systemic review of long term effects of advice to reduce dietary salt in adults. *BMJ.* **325**: 628–32.

Insua JT, Sacks HS, Lau TS et al.(1994) Drug treatment of hypertension in the elderly: a meta-analysis. *Ann Intern Med.* **121**: 355–62.

Joint National Congress on Detection, Evaluation and Treatment of High Blood Pressure (1993) Fifth Report (JNC V). *Arch Intern Med.* **153**: 154–83.

Kaplan NM (1994) Ethnic aspects of hypertension. *Lancet.* **344**: 450–2.

Khattar RS, Swales JD, Senior S and Lahiri A (2000) Racial variation in cardiovascular morbidity and mortality in essential hypertension. *Heart.* **83**: 267–71.

Kostis JB, Davis BR, Cutler J et al. (1997) Prevention of heart failure by antihypertensive drug treatment in older persons with isolated systolic hypertension. SHEP Cooperative Research Group. *JAMA.* **278**: 212–16.

Lever AF and Ramsay LE (1995) Treatment of hypertension in the elderly. *J Hypertens.* **13**: 571–9.

Littenburg B and Wolfberg C (1998) Pseudohypertension masquerading as malignant hypertension. Case report and review of the literature. *Am J Med.* **84**: 539–42.

McKeigue PM, Marmot MG, Adelstein AM et al.(1985) Diet and risk factors for coronary artery disease in Asians in northwest London. *Lancet.* **ii**: 1086–90.

McKeigue PM, Marmot MG, Court YDS et al. (1988) Diabetes, hyperinsulinaemia and coronary risk factors in Bangladeshi in East London. *Br Heart J.* **60**: 390–6.

McKeigue PM, Shah B and Marmot MG (1991) Relation of central obesity and insulin resistance with high diabetes prevalence and cardiovascular risk in South Asians. *Lancet.* **337**: 382–6.

Medical Research Council (1992) Trial of treatment of hypertension in older adults: principal results. MRC Working Party. *BMJ.* **304**: 405–12.

Messerli FH, Grossman E and Goldbourt U (1998) Are beta-blockers efficacious as first-line therapy for hypertension in the elderly? A systematic review. *JAMA.* **279**: 1903–7.

Mulrow CD, Cornell JA, Herrera CR, Kadri A, Farnett L and Aguilar C (1994) Hypertension in the elderly. Implications and generalizability of randomized trials. *JAMA.* **272**: 1932–8.

Pfeffer MA, Braunwald E, Moye LA et al. (1992) Effect of Captopril on mortality and morbidity in patients with left ventricular dysfunction after myocardial infarction. Results of the Survival And Ventricular Enlargement trial. The SAVE Investigators. *N Engl J Med.* **327**: 669–77.

PROGRESS Collaborative Group (2001) Randomised trial of a Perindopril-based blood pressure lowering regimen among 6,105 patients with prior stroke or transient ischaemic attack. *Lancet.* **358**: 1033–41.

Ramsey LE, Williams B, Johanston DG et al. (1999) British Hypertensive Society guidelines for hypertensive management 1999: a summary. *BMJ.* **319**: 630–5.

SHEP Cooperative Research Group (1991) Prevention of stroke by antihypertensive drug treatment in older persons with isolated systolic hypertension. Final results of the Systolic Hypertension in the Elderly Program (SHEP). *JAMA.* **265**: 3255–64.

Skoog I, Lernfelt B, Landahl S et al. (1996) 15-year longitudinal study of blood pressure and dementia. *Lancet.* **347**: 1141–5.

Staessen JA, Fagard R, Thijs L et al. (1997) Randomised double-blind comparison of placebo and active treatment for older patients with isolated systolic hypertension. The Systolic Hypertension in Europe (Syst-Eur) Trial Investigators. *Lancet.* **350**: 757–64.

UK Prospective Diabetes Study Group (1998) Tight blood pressure control and risk of macrovascular and microvascular complications in type 2 diabetes: UKPDS 38. *BMJ.* **317**: 703–13.

Whelton PK, Appel LJ, Espeland MA et al. (1998) Sodium reduction and weight loss in the treatment of hypertension in older persons: a randomized controlled trial of nonpharmacologic interventions in the elderly (TONE). TONE Collaborative Research Group. *JAMA.* **279**: 839–46.

Williams B, Poulter NR, Brown MJ et al. (2004) Guidelines for management of hypertension: report of the fourth working party of the British Hypertension Society, 2004 – BHS IV. *J Hum Hypertens.* **18**: 139–85.

Wood D, Durrington P, Poulter N et al. on behalf of the British Cardiac Society, British Hyperlipidaemia Association, British Hypertension Society, and Pearce KA, Furberg CD, Rushing J (1995) Does antihypertensive treatment of the elderly prevent cardiovascular events or prolong life? A meta-analysis of hypertension treatment trials. *Arch Fam Med*. **4**: 943–9.

Chapter 7

Cardiovascular disease

Introduction

Coronary heart disease (CHD) is the most common cause of mortality in the Western hemisphere. Its incidence increases with age and the vast majority of patients suffering with CHD are elderly. The elderly constitute the majority of patients who develop myocardial infarction and a major proportion of the patients who die of this pathology. Over the past three decades there has been a reduction in mortality from cardiovascular diseases in most Western countries but CHD remains the main cause of death.

In the UK, people of Indo-Asian origin have 40% higher mortality from CHD compared with the white population. In Indo-Asians the onset of disease is early and the mortality is higher, suggesting a significant role of ethnicity in the development of CHD. The increased risk for CHD not only applies to first-generation immigrant Indo-Asians but extends to subsequent generations. The high risk is also noticeable in Indo-Asian females, in contrast to the relative immunity from CHD noted in Western women. Nonetheless, ethnic minorities have been under-represented in clinical trials of ischaemic heart disease.

The increased risk for ischaemic heart disease in Indo-Asians is not a new phenomenon and is not specific to their community in the UK. First recognised over 40 years ago, this trend has been observed around the globe. The differences are more pronounced at a younger age. This variability in cardiovascular disease based on ethnic differences has shed new light on the aetiology of ischaemic heart disease and has helped not only ethnic minorities but every patient with CHD.

Prevalence

The *Health Survey for England* (Primatesta 1999) showed stark differences between Indo-Asians and the general population, with Indo-Asians showing higher rates for coronary heart disease and stroke. There were differences within the Indo-Asian community, with the Pakistani and Bangladeshi communities showing far higher rates for these pathologies than the Indian. Pakistani and Bangladeshi communities showed a five times higher rate for diabetes than the Caucasian population, whereas the rate for the Indian community was three times higher. Contrary to the trend in the general population, higher levels of CHD and stroke were noted among the non-manual social class in the Indo-Asian community.

Indo-Asians and coronary heart disease

Despite the diversity, the increased risk of CHD is shared by all ethnic groups of Indo-Asian origin. There are several hallmarks of CHD in this community, with early presentation, more extensive atheroma and higher incidence of triple vessel disease. The rate of myocardial infarction is five times greater and the highest mortality is observed in Muslim males, particularly in the third and fourth decades. They have a lower ejection fraction and impaired left ventricular functions. Overall, the mortality from CHD in this group is 1.5 times higher than the general population. While mortality from CHD is decreasing in the white UK population, this trend is far less pronounced in the Indo-Asian community.

Reliable data on CHD from the Indian subcontinent are sparse. It seems that the Indo-Asians living in the UK may have a greater risk of CHD as compared with their counterparts in the Indian subcontinent. In the Indian subcontinent the incidence of CHD varies greatly depending upon the socio-economic background and geographical distribution of the population. Therefore it is not possible to compare Indo-Asians in the UK with the native population of the Indian subcontinent.

Following their arrival in developed countries, migrants from the Indian subcontinent acquire unfavourable risks for developing CHD. Though some of these risk factors may be secondary to exposure to a Western lifestyle, the evidence for this being the main factor is lacking. It is plausible that the Indo-Asian population has a genetic predisposition to atherosclerotic and antithrombotic risk factors. Migration to the West or change to a Western lifestyle may be a catalyst, thus unmasking these risks and hence increasing the probability for developing CHD.

Atherosclerosis in Indo-Asians

Atherosclerosis is a chronic inflammatory condition. Atherosclerotic plaque rupture and subsequent thrombosis lead to an acute clinical event. There are differences in the composition and stability of atherosclerotic plaques in Indo-Asians which may in part be responsible for the high morbidity and mortality from vascular disease in this section of the population. Indo-Asians have severe, non-discrete plaques and triple vessel disease. Differences in the composition of these plaques may go some way to explaining the increased incidence of myocardial infarction in Indo-Asians. In conjunction with other risk factors, instability of atherosclerotic plaques may be partially responsible for high morbidity and mortality from vascular disease.

Risk factors for coronary heart disease

The high incidence of CHD in Indo-Asians could not be explained purely on the basis of conventional risk factors such as hypertension, smoking and total cholesterol concentration. The prevalence of some of these classic risk factors is lower in the Indo-Asian community, they vary greatly within this population and do not provide a plausible explanation for the increased incidence of CHD (Box 7.1). On the other hand, high triglycerides, low HDL-cholesterol, high homocysteine levels, central obesity, high prevalence of insulin resistance syndrome and diabetes may provide a more plausible explanation for the increase in CHD. Adverse thrombogenic factors further augment the risk for CHD. Unlike conventional risk factors, most Indo-Asian communities share these risk factors.

Indo-Asians are more prone to complications secondary to ischaemic heart disease. Thus it is plausible that a lower threshold for intervention is needed for initiating investigations and treatment in these groups. Clinical evidence from studies predominantly in the Caucasian population could not be directly extrapolated to the Indo-Asian population living in the UK or in their native countries.

Box 7.1 Risk factors for coronary heart disease in Indo-Asians

---

- Hyperinsulinaemia
- High fasting triglycerides
- Low HDL
- High fibrinogen
- Elevated plasminogen activator inhibitor-1
- Increased homocysteine
- Increased C-reactive protein (CRP)
- High lipoprotein (Lp)(a)
- Impaired endothelial functions
- Unstable atherosclerotic plaques

Insulin resistance syndrome

It is well recognised that cardiovascular risk factors, including Type 2 diabetes, dyslipidaemia, hypertension and central obesity, may co-exist in the same patient. In the Indo-Asian population, insulin resistance syndrome may provide some clues to the deranged metabolic profile. The hallmarks of this syndrome include central obesity with a waist-to-hip ratio of >1.0 in men and 0.85 in women, high fasting triglyceride >1.5 mmol/L, low HDL-cholesterol <1.0 mmol/L, fasting glucose of >7.0 mmol/L and hyperinsulinism. Hyperinsulinaemia may in part be responsible for proliferation of vascular smooth muscle cells or could exert influence on the prothrombotic factors, including the concentration of fibrinogen, plasminogen activator I and factor VIIc. It is important to recognise that Indo-Asians exhibit evidence of insulin resistance at an early age and the association of insulin resistance and obesity may express itself at a lower level of obesity.

The predisposing factors for insulin resistance syndrome are not clear but genetic factors plus urban migration or migration with adoption of a Western lifestyle seem to be important predisposing factors. Poor foetal growth and low birth weight have been shown to have an association with insulin resistance.

There are some modifiable influences for prevention of insulin resistance which include exercise and restricting carbohydrate and caloric intake. Weight loss by restricting fats is important and achievable. In Indo-Asians, fat consumption can be reduced effectively but needs involvement of all the members of the extended household. Although obesity is a strong risk factor for insulin resistance syndrome, the syndrome could also be encountered in non-obese people.

Dyslipidaemia

The role of lipids in the pathogenesis of CHD is well established. Indo-Asians have generally low total cholesterol as compared with the white population but have low HDL-cholesterol and higher fasting triglycerides. An increase in lipoprotein (a) in Indo-Asians may be genetically determined and constitutes an adverse risk for CHD.

Analysis of many randomised control trials showed benefit in older patients for both primary and secondary prevention. Hence age alone should not be the basis for withholding HMG Co-A reductase therapy in older people.

There is no single definition for the Indo-Asian diet as there is vast variation with thousands of different social and cultural groups. Although the total fat content of the Indo-Asian diet is no different from that of the general white population, the ratio of polyunsaturated to saturated fat is higher.

There are ample data to suggest that CHD is preventable by reducing modifiable risk factors. The high risks associated with dyslipidaemia and other associated factors in Indo-Asians may be underestimated when compared with the Caucasian population. As Indo-Asians have different risk factors, guidelines created predominantly for the white populations of the UK and USA should not be rigidly applied to Indo-Asians. A lower threshold for intervention for lipid lowering should be considered. In Indo-Asians total cholesterol should be less than 4 mmol/L, LDL cholesterol 2.5 mmol/L, triglycerides 1.5 mmoL/s and HDL should be more than 1 mmol/L. These recommendations are based on non-migrant low-risk groups. Values for treating dyslipidaemia in the Western population would be misleading in Indo-Asians. Statins should be used early in high-risk patients for both lowering total cholesterol and for treating mild triglyceridaemia.

Pro-coagulant state

There are some independent markers for the pro-coagulant state which constitutes a risk factor for cardiovascular disease. These factors include plasminogen activator inhibitor-1 (PAI-1), tissue plasminogen activator (t-PA) and to some extent fibrinogen, von Willebrand factor (vWF) and factor VII:C.

PAI-1 in Indo-Asians has been shown to be higher than in the general population and fibrinogen has also been reported to be higher in Indo-Asians. Fibrinogen is higher in Indo-Asian patients with CHD and diabetes as compared with patients with just CHD. The level of factor VII:C is recorded to be lower in Indo-Asians as compared with the white population. These factors on their own or in combination may provide a possible link with increased cardiovascular disease in Indo-Asians. However, their precise role in the pro-coagulant state in Indo-Asians is less clear. There is evidence that insulin resistance syndrome and diabetes are associated with these risk factors.

Homocysteine

Homocysteine is a sulphur-containing amino acid. Plasma homocysteine is a well-recognised risk factor for coronary artery disease (CAD). Approximately 40% of patients with vascular disease have homocysteine concentrations above the 80th centile of normal. Studies have shown that even a small rise in homocysteine leads to a large increase in the risk for CAD.

Plasma concentration of homocysteine is dependent upon multiple factors including genetic constitution, vitamins B6 and B12 and folic acid levels.

Elevated plasma homocysteine has been proven to be a risk factor for CAD in Indo-Asians and may be in part responsible for the increased risk of CAD in this community. Studies have shown fasting homocysteine levels up to 6% higher in Indo-Asians living in the UK as compared with the European population.

Significantly reduced concentrations of vitamin B12 and folate have also been noted in Indo-Asians and may be contributory factors in elevated plasma homocysteine. Methods of preparing food in the Indo-Asian community can include prolonged cooking of vegetables on high heat which could result in destruction of up to 90% of the folate content. Apart from dietary factors, homocysteine rises along with creatinine and renal impairment is not uncommon in Indo-Asians.

As high homocysteine could be a result of reduced vitamin B12 and folate intake, some authorities have recommended vitamin and folate supplementation to reduce the risk of CAD in the Indo-Asian community. However, there is no evidence to show an impact of lowering homocysteine on CAD in the longitudinal studies.

Hypertension

The prevalence of hypertension increases to over 50% in people over 65 years of age living in the developed world. Hypertension is one of the main modifiable risk factors for CHD.

Hypertension is more common in Indo-Asians as compared with the Caucasian population and has a bearing on the incidence of CHD in this community. Multiple factors, including social, economic, genetic and cultural influences, effects of migration, change in environment and dietary changes, may be responsible. Hypertension combined with the features of the insulin resistance syndrome increases the risk for CHD several-fold.

As hypertension is an important modifiable risk factor, it is recommended that Indo-Asians should have blood pressure below 140 mmHg systolic and 85 mmHg diastolic, similar to the standard for the non-migrant population.

Physical activity

Exercise has an inverse relationship with obesity and risk for cardiovascular disease. Exercise of 30 minutes a day has been shown to reduce cardiovascular risks. Indo-Asians who are more active have lower BMI and lower concentrations of insulin and triglycerides. Regrettably the Indo-Asian population in the UK has a lower level of physical activity than the white population, which increases their risk for CHD. More detailed reference to this effect has been made in Chapter 3. Old age is associated with altered endothelial function and, in Indo-Asians with insulin resistance syndrome, exercise has a beneficial effect.

Diet and obesity

Obesity is related to CHD, insulin resistance and diabetes. Overall obesity is low in Indo-Asians as compared with the general population but they have a higher fat content and more subcutaneous fat. Thus it is important to remember that the terminology adopted to describe obesity in the Western population will be inappropriate for ethnic minorities. The increased central obesity makes the usual means of defining obesity invalid. There is no single cut-off point for all Asians but recently the World Health Organization has recommended a lower BMI as desirable for public health actions in Indo-Asians. More detailed reference to this effect and the BMI has been made in Chapter 3.

The high risk for CHD in Indo-Asians may be linked to dietary factors such as consumption of *ghee* (clarified butter). Increased consumption of *ghee*, raised levels of trans fatty acids and low linoleic acid in fatty tissue could lead to increased risk for CHD. However, polyunsaturated fat consumption is higher and fat in food as a percentage of the total calorie intake is low as compared with the white population. The diet of Indo-Asians is carbohydrate rich so the advice given to the white population to follow a high carbohydrate diet may be ineffective. In the Indo-Asian population restriction of calories and consumption of low-fat foods may be more appropriate. A detailed account of the Indo-Asian diet is given in Chapter 3.

Tobacco and smoking

Smoking is a major risk factor for CHD, insulin resistance, glucose metabolism and haemostatic functions. Smoking is widespread in all Asian communities with the exception of the Sikhs. The prevalence of cigarette smoking decreases with age but constitutes a strong risk factor for ischaemic heart disease. More detailed reference to this effect has been made in Chapter 3.

Inflammatory response

Apart from the traditional risk factors for CHD, researchers are looking for evidence in other areas. Inflammation, infection and endothelial functions are being explored in an attempt to clarify the increased incidence for CHD in Indo-Asians. Elevated C-reactive protein (CRP) is an independent risk factor for CHD. CRP concentrations have been noted to be elevated in Indo-Asians and are related to fasting and post-load insulin.

Other risk factors

Lipoprotein (Lp) (a) is largely genetically determined and has been shown to be associated with up to nine times increased risk of CHD, particularly in the presence of raised low-density lipoproteins. Levels of Lp(a) have been shown to be higher in Indo-Asians.

Impaired vascular endothelial functions have been noticed in Indo-Asians as compared with Europeans and may have a part to play in the development of CHD. Depression has also been linked with ischaemic heart disease and is associated with increased mortality.

Ageing and coronary heart disease

Old age brings some physiological changes in the cardiovascular system which increase the chances of CHD in the elderly. These factors include decreased vascular compliance, increased afterload, decreased endothelial responsiveness and decreased responsiveness to beta-adrenergic stimulation. Cardiac ageing, on the other hand, is associated with prolonged contraction and decreased early ventricular diastolic filling. These changes cause elderly patients to develop early dyspnoeic symptoms secondary to ischaemic insult or cardiac arrhythmias.

The mortality and risks of complications associated with myocardial infarction are much higher in the elderly as compared with the younger age group. There are limitations to thrombolysis in old age, with many patients not being eligible for thrombolytic therapy. Complication rates are also higher and myocardial rupture is common. Non-Q wave infarction is more common in the elderly and is associated with increased risks. If ischaemic symptoms persist after non-Q wave myocardial infarction, then early coronary angiography and revascularisation are recommended regardless of age.

There is clear evidence that elderly patients benefit as much from risk reduction as younger patients. Considering the high absolute risk in this population, the benefit is higher in this group. These benefits may be even higher when dealing with elders of Indo-Asian origin. Weight and height decrease with age and this is an important issue to remember when dealing with elders of Indo-Asians origin.

Anatomical differences in coronary arteries

Indo-Asians have generally smaller coronary arteries as compared with Europeans. Though this is in line with the small stature of Indo-Asians, it does pose some difficulties during invasive procedures. Smaller vessels, along with more extensive and diffuse disease, make good results more difficult to achieve. The angiographic pattern in Indo-Asians is similar to the one observed in diabetic patients.

Management of coronary heart disease

Managing CHD in older patients is complex and challenging. The principles of CHD management in Indo-Asian patients are similar to those for European patients. Silent ischaemia is common and can affect one-third of patients over the age of 70. Therefore, a classic history of CHD may not be as reliable in the elderly as in younger age groups. Decreased perception of pain, decreased exercise capacity or associated pathology such as osteo-arthritis may limit a patient's mobility to the extent that they do not experience symptoms and hence CHD may not surface. In many patients dyspnoea may be the first symptom associated with CHD, rather than chest pain. In elders of Indo-Asian origin these problems could be compounded by poor communication. The true incidence of silent ischaemia in this cohort is not known and no study has addressed the presentation of CHD in ethnic elders from Indo-Asia.

Cardiac rehabilitation is an essential aspect of management following a myocardial infarction. It has been proven to be safe and help preserve functional abilities in older patients after myocardial infarction. In Indo-Asian patients there would be a high need for this service but many patients will require information in their own language. Projects targeted to specific communities may have more success in influencing patients and their therapy.

Investigations

A full blood count, renal functions, random glucose, serum lipids, thyroid function test, an electrocardiogram and a chest X-ray should be requested on the first visit. Investigations required for diagnostic purposes should include general investigations to exclude pathologies such as thyrotoxicosis or anaemia.

An exercise stress test is useful in clarifying the diagnosis but there are limitations in older people which need addressing. Many elderly patients are unable to exercise due to disabilities such as arthritis or chronic obstructive airway disease. A high incidence of abnormal electrocardiograms secondary to bundle branch block, left ventricular hypertrophy and a digoxin effect may decrease the predictive accuracy of a positive test. It should be borne in mind that the predictive accuracy of a negative test is low in a cohort with a high prevalence of the disease.

A pharmacological stress test is another practical method in elderly patients. Pharmacological agents such as dobutamine or adenosine could be used in conjunction with isotopic studies or with stress echo for diagnostic purposes or to support other investigations. However, their use may be limited by their availability in many centres. Elderly patients find it difficult to travel long distances for these investigations and could be disadvantaged by the lack of availability of cardiovascular diagnostic services in their local hospitals.

Medications for coronary heart disease

Over 50% of prescriptions are for patients 65 years and over. Older patients benefit as much as young from secondary and primary prevention treatment. Medications offer functional independence, improved quality of life and enhanced life expectancy in cardiovascular disease. However, the elderly are at particular risk with medications. Physiology of ageing, increased co-morbidity, high incidence of adverse drug reactions and problems with drug compliance, compounded with problems of ethnicity, make treatment in Indo-Asian elders particularly challenging. Despite all these difficulties, medication should not be withheld from elderly patients on the basis of age alone.

Indo-Asians respond to medications in the same manner as the Caucasian population. However, they have a predisposition to insulin resistance syndrome with high triglycerides, low HDL-cholesterol and central obesity plus high prevalence of diabetes. These issues should be considered when choosing a treatment option. Certain drugs create a susceptibility to an undesirable lipid profile and can worsen this metabolic syndrome which may negate any beneficial effect of their protective action on the cardiovascular system. There is evidence that treatment with diuretics and beta-blockers further increases insulin resistance which in turn raises the risk of developing Type 2 diabetes or impaired glucose tolerance, both of which are associated with increased risk of CHD. However, it remains unclear whether diabetes mellitus induced by beta-blockers or thiazide diuretics is associated with increased risk of CHD.

When treating Indo-Asian patients, it would be advantageous to avoid thiazide diuretics or beta-blockers as first-line therapy for hypertension and, if alternatives exist, to explore them before using these medications. Drugs which improve the metabolic imbalance should be the first choice. The beneficial effects of ACE inhibitors and angiotensin II receptor antagonists may be more desirable in Indo-Asians with ischaemic heart disease, along with beta-blockers. ACE inhibitors have other benefits beyond reduction of blood pressure. Other examples would be pioglitazone in diabetes and the use of alpha-blockers in hypertension. Most other drugs used for CHD have neutral effect on lipids and glucose metabolism and their use should be similar to the Caucasian population.

Other drugs which may be used for patients with CHD include sublingual or oral nitrates. Calcium channel blockers and potassium channel regulators may be used in selected patients. ACEI are beneficial in CHD and should be considered for all elderly patients. Use of aspirin is essential for all patients unless there is a specific contraindication and glycoprotein IIb/IIIa inhibitors should be considered for selected patients. Unfractionated heparin or low molecular weight heparin is essential for patients with acute coronary syndrome. There is increased risk of bleeding complications but the benefit outweighs any concerns.

Use of statins in elderly patients

There has been fierce debate regarding the use of lipid-lowering therapy in older patients with ischaemic heart disease. The Prospective Study of Pravastatin in the Elderly at Risk (PROSPER) trial has shown clear benefits of statin therapy on vascular risk factors in the elderly. The trial showed that patients with the lowest baseline high-density lipoproteins gained most from statin therapy. This has implications for the treatment of Indo-Asian patients. Hence, there is little doubt that elderly patients benefit from aggressive lipid lowering with statins. Early introduction of statins after myocardial infarction irrespective of serum lipids is now a common recommendation.

Interventional cardiology

In patients with CHD, percutaneous transluminal coronary angioplasty (PTCA) could be a suitable option for those with contraindications to surgery and who have continued symptoms despite adequate medical therapy. With newer techniques and the advent of coronary artery stents, the success rate has improved.

Review of the current published literature suggests that elderly patients benefit from PTCA but have a higher incidence of target lesion calcification and small reference vessel diameter. Bleeding complications and mortality in some studies were high and the hospital stay was longer. However, elderly patients have a high co-morbidity which influences the outcome after PTCA. Poor cardiac functions, diabetes or renal failure may play a part in poor outcomes. There are few outcome data in elderly patients of Indo-Asian origin.

Coronary artery bypass surgery

Innovations in the field of cardiovascular surgery and anaesthesia mean that a significant number of elderly patients can now be considered for coronary artery bypass graft. As a result, the vast majority of patients undergoing coronary artery bypass graft are elderly. For surgical intervention, the risks increase steeply in patients over the age of 80. Surgery is usually the last option for these patients and it is not surprising that there is a higher incidence of complications and mortality in this group.

Factors which serve as markers for operative mortality in older patients include prior cardiac bypass surgery, female sex, peripheral vascular disease, diabetes, renal failure, peripheral vascular disease and, most importantly, left ventricular systolic functions. Advanced old age is also a factor for poor outcome and for postoperative stroke and cognitive decline after surgery.

Prognosis

Determining prognosis in elderly patients with stable CHD is difficult. It mainly depends upon associated factors such as left ventricular functions and the extent of vascular disease. Absence of symptoms is an unreliable guide to evaluating the extent of disease.

Heart failure in Indo-Asian patients

Like many other areas, information on heart failure in the Indo-Asian population is lacking. Hypertension, ischaemic heart disease, insulin resistance and diabetes are more common in Indo-Asians and may contribute to the development of heart failure. A UK study of heart failure showed that compared with white patients, Indo-Asian patients admitted to hospital for the first time with heart failure were younger and had diabetes or myocardial infarction. However, outcomes were similar for the two groups and mortality was lower in the Indo-Asian group. These observations clearly show the importance of further studies in Indo-Asians.

Peripheral vascular disease in Indo-Asians

There are few scientific data on the ethnic differences in peripheral vascular disease (PVD). However, the limited data which exist are interesting as, despite higher risk factors for CHD, the incidence for PVD is low in Indo-

Asians compared with Europeans. More research is required to clarify this discrepancy.

Ischaemic heart disease, driving and the DVLA

The basic information on driving and DVLA rules have been detailed in Chapter 5. Ischaemic heart disease and rules for driving are available from the DVLA guide to current medical standards of fitness to drive. Current recommendations are that for angina (Group I) it is not a legal requirement to notify the DVLA. Patients with angina should cease driving when symptoms occur at rest or while the patient is driving. Driving can resume with symptom control. For angioplasty (Group I) it is not a legal requirement to notify the DVLA. Patients should cease driving for at least one week. For patients with acute coronary syndrome (Group I), it is not a legal requirement to notify the DVLA. Driving must cease after myocardial infarction (MI) for at least four weeks. Patients can drive thereafter if there are no disqualifying conditions. Following a non-ST elevation MI, driving can restart after one week following successful angioplasty provided there is no other disqualifying condition. It is recommended that patients should consult the DVLA for advice as the recommendations are subject to change.

Access to healthcare and coronary heart disease

Indo-Asians are less likely to receive appropriate care for CHD. This holds true for acute as well as chronic coronary artery disease. They have to wait significantly longer to be seen by specialist services as compared with the general population. Though they have high risks, they are less likely to receive diagnostic and interventional procedures. These trends are particularly prominent in elders of Indo-Asian origin, women and patients from a deprived social background.

The reasons for this inequality may be multifactorial. The history may be deemed atypical in these patients and the interpretation of symptoms may be difficult for healthcare workers. Difficulties in finding the right word for the given symptom or responding in a different manner to a standard question may lead to delay in accurate diagnosis.

The concept of long-term medications for chronic disease such as dyslipidaemia and hypertension is relatively new to the elderly Indo-Asian population. Reasons for taking medicine may not be understood clearly by some patients and poor compliance may contribute to poor outcome.

Prevention of cardiovascular disease in Indo-Asians

There is little doubt that with adequate early intervention, CHD is not only reducible but preventable. Many relatives of patients with CHD will have dyslipidaemia and hence increased risk for CHD. Targeting and screening of first-degree relatives can be an important preventive strategy.

Indo-Asians in the UK, being a heterogeneous group, require a more targeted approach. The risk factors may be different in different ethnic communities. As a general rule, anti-smoking and tobacco chewing campaigns should be directed toward Bangladeshis and not at Sikh communities. Dietary advice is important and needs to be part of any campaign aimed at reducing CHD. Religious festivals and rituals may be important in directing these campaigns when communities are more receptive to advice and change. The best example of this is the month of Ramadan when Muslims are most likely to accept anti-smoking or dietary advice.

Diet and the content of food consumed may differ from one community to another and skilled dieticians well versed in the requirements of the ethnic group would be needed to provide advice.

Indo-Asians with a strong family history, established risk factors and existing CHD are a high-risk group. The need is for urgent multidisciplinary intervention with a holistic approach rather than tackling a single risk factor. Teams of physicians, nurses, dieticians and other health workers who deal with Indo-Asian patients need knowledge of the sociocultural and religious background of their targeted population. Availability of information and education are the foundations of any preventive programme (Box 7.2).

Box 7.2 Management issues for treating elderly patients

- High use of medical facilities
- High use of diagnostic facilities
- Increased use of pharmacological resources
- Longer length of hospital stay
- Increased use of rehabilitation and social service resources

---

There is a need for educational programmes to involve schools, cultural centres and religious venues where large numbers of Indo-Asians gather on a regular basis. A targeted and focused approach for each individual group may prove more fruitful. Ethnic minority religious organisations and community leaders need to share responsibility and work with their local authorities and hospitals to improve awareness of CHD in Indo-Asians.

Conclusion

Ethnicity plays a significant role in the development of CHD. Elders of Indo-Asian origin have higher risk factors and hence are more at risk. There is some evidence to suggest that as a group they are at a disadvantage when it comes to accurate diagnosis, investigations and intervention. Regrettably, there are no studies which have looked specifically at Indo-Asian elders as a group. The medical knowledge for treating this group is based mainly on studies of European patients or on only partial data from the Indo-Asian community.

More research is required to explore specific risks, clinical course and prognosis of CHD in Indo-Asians. Special attention should be given to disease mechanisms which may explain many aspects of CHD that are still shrouded in mystery. Research is also needed to explore dietary and social practices and disease presentation in Indo-Asians. The impact of CHD on future generations will be a challenge facing health planners and researchers alike.

Audit has a part to play in primary and secondary care settings. Looking at the uptake of preventive and diagnostic services is crucial to any programme. Audits will be essential to monitor access to specialist services for ethnic minorities, and especially ethnic elders, along with invasive investigations and treatment.

The risks for CHD in Indo-Asians are high and merit early intervention. Guidelines based on the predominantly white population of the UK, Europe and North America should not be rigidly applied when dealing with Indo-Asian communities, in whom the threshold for intervention should be low. Early and accurate diagnosis of CHD in this group is essential. Awareness of CHD and education on prevention are essential to prevent cardiac problems in the Indo-Asian community overwhelming the cardiac services in future.

Involvement of the community is essential for the success of any project. The responsibility for improving the health needs of a community should be shared by the leaders of minority groups, religious figures, social organisations and local health authorities. Sharing local experiences and successful models of care with other national agencies and organisations would be desirable but needs planning and foresight. Conventional models of service delivery do not cater for the needs of all ethnic minorities and rigid blanket programmes targeted towards ethnic minorities are doomed to failure.

In the UK the time is ripe for politicians and health planners to invest in preventive strategies targeting individual Indo-Asian communities. A modest investment now may prevent a large burden on health resources in future and much suffering and pain in the Indo-Asian community.

Further reading

American Heart Association (1994) *Heart and Stroke Facts.* 1994 Statistical Supplement. American Heart Association, Dallas, Texas.

Anand SS, Yousaf S, Vuksan V et al. (2000) Difference in risk factors, atherosclerosis and cardiovascular disease between ethnic groups in Canada: the Study of Health Assessment and Risk in Ethnic Groups (SHARE). *Lancet.* **356**: 279–84.

Ang PC, Farouque HM, Harper RW, Meredith IT (2000) Percutaneous coronary intervention in the elderly: a comparison of procedural and clinical outcomes between the eighth and ninth decade. *J Invas Cardiol.* **12**: 488–92.

Balarajan R (1991) Ethnic differences in mortality from ischaemic heart disease and cerebrovascular disease in England and Wales. *BMJ.* **302**: 560–4.

Balarajan R (1996) Ethnicity and variations in mortality from coronary heart disease. *Health Trends.* **28**: 45.

Baralajan R and Soni Raleigh V (1995) *Ethnicity and Health in England.* HMSO, London.

Bass EB, Follansbee WP and Orchard TJ (1981) Comparison of supplemented Rose Questionnaire to exercise tallium testing in men and in women. *J Clin Epidemiol.* **42**: 385–94.

Batchelor WB, Anstron KJ, Mulbair LH et al. (2001) Contemporary outcome trends in the elderly undergoing percutaneous coronary intervention: results in 7472 octogenarians. *J Am Coll Cardiol*. **36**: 723–30.

Bhatnagar D, Anand IS, Durrington PN et al. (1995) Coronary risk factors in people from Indian subcontinent living in west London and their siblings in India. *Lancet*. **345**: 405–9.

Bhopal R, Unwin N, Whites M et al. (1999) Heterogeneity of coronary heart disease risk factors in Indians, Pakistani, Bangladeshi and European origin population: cross sectional study. *BMJ*. **319**: 215–20.

Blackburn H, Keys A and Simonson E (1960) The electrocardiogram in population studies: a classification system. *Circulation*. **21**: 1160–75.

Blackwalder WC, Kagan A, Gordon T and Rhoads GG (1981) Comparisons of methods for diagnosing angina pectoris: the Honolulu heart study. *Int J Epidemiol*. **10**: 211–15.

Chambers JC, Obeid OA, Refsum H et al. (2000) Plasma homocysteine concentration and risk of coronary heart disease in UK Indian Asian and European men. *Lancet*. **355**: 523–7.

Dhawan J and Bray CL (1994) Angiographic comparison of coronary artery disease between Asians and Caucasians. *Postgrad Med J*. **70**: 625–30.

Drever F and Whitehead M (1997) *Health Inequalities*. Decennial supplement. Series DS No.15. Stationery Office, London.

Feder G, Crook AM, Magee P et al. (2002) Ethnic differences in invasive management of coronary disease: prospective cohort study of patients undergoing angiography. *BMJ*. **324**: 511–16.

Fischbaker CM, Bhopal R, White M, Unwin N and Alberti KGM (2000) The comparative performance of the Rose Angina questionnaire in South Asian population. *J Epidemiol Community Health*. **54**: 786.

Heart Protection Study Collaborative Group (2002) The MRC/BHF Heart Protection Study of cholesterol lowering with simvastatin in 20,536 high-risk individuals: a randomized placebo controlled trial. *Lancet*. **360**: 7–22.

Hughes LO, Raval U and Raftery EB (1980) First myocardial infarction in Asians and white men. *BMJ*. **298**: 1345–50.

Juhan-Vague I, Alessi MC and Vague P (1990) Thrombogenic and fibrinolytic factors and cardiovascular risk in non-insulin dependent diabetes mellitus. *Ann Med*. **28**: 371–80.

Juhan-Vague I, Thompson SG and Jesperson J (1993) Involvement of the hemostastic system in the insulin resistance syndrome. A study of 1500 patients with angina pectoris. The ECAT Angina Pectoris Study Group. *Arterioscler Thromb*. **13**: 1865–73.

Kain K, Catto AJ and Grant PJ (2001) Impaired fibrinolysis and increased fibrinogen levels in South Asian subjects. *Atherosclerosis*. **156**: 457–61.

Knight TM, Smith Z, Whittles A et al. (1992) Insulin resistance, diabetes and risk markers for ischaemic heart disease in Asian men and non-Asian in Bradford. *Br Heart J*. **67**: 343–50.

Lanza GA (2004) Ethnic variations in acute coronary syndrome. *Heart*. **90**: 595–7.

Lear JT, Lawrence IG, Pohl JEF and Burden AC (1994) Myocardial infarction and thrombolysis: a comparison of the Indian and European populations on a coronary care unit. *J Roy Coll Phys London*. **28(2)**: 143–7.

Lee J, Heng D, Chia KS, Chew SK, Tan BY and Hughes K (2001) Risk factors and incident coronary heart disease in Chinese, Malays and Asian Indian males: the Singapore cardiovascular cohort study. *Int J Epidemiol.* **30**: 983–8.

Lusis AJ (2000) Atherosclerosis. *Nature.* **407**: 233–41.

Mather HM and Keen H (1985) The Southall diabetes survey: prevalence of diabetes in Asians and Europeans. *BMJ.* **291**: 1081–4.

McKeighue PM, Miller G and Marmot MG (1989) Coronary artery disease in South Asians overseas – a review. *J Clin Epidemiol.* **42**: 597–609.

McKeighue PM, Shah B and Marmot MG (1991) Relation of central obesity and insulin resistance with high diabetes prevalence and cardiovascular risk in South Asians. *Lancet.* **337**: 382–6.

McKeighue PM, Marmot MG, Syndercombe Court YD, Cottier DE, Rahman S and Reimersma RA (1997) Diabetes, hyperinsulinaemia and coronary risk factors in Bangladeshi in east London. *Heart.* **78**: 63–72.

Miller GJ, Beckles GL, Maude GH et al. (1989) Ethnicity and other characteristics predictive of coronary heart disease in a developing community: principal results of the St James survey, Trinidad. *Int J Epidemiol.* **18**: 808.

Muhktar HT and Littler WA (1995) Survival after acute myocardial infarction in Asian and white patients in Birmingham. *Br Heart J.* **73**: 122–4.

Nazroo JY (1997) *The Health of Britain's Ethnic Minorities: Findings from a National Survey.* Policy Studies Institute, London.

Obaid OA, Mannan N, Perry G, Iles RA and Boucher BJ (1998) Homocysteine and folate deficiency in healthy East London Bangladeshis. *Lancet.* **352**: 1829–30.

Peterson ED, Cowper PA, Jollis JG et al. (1995) Outcome of coronary artery bypass graft surgery in 24,461 patients aged 80 years or older. *Circulation.* **92**: 85–91.

Primatesta P (1999) Relationship of CVD to risk factors and socio-demographic factors. In: B Erens, P Primatesta (eds) *Health Survey for England: Cardiovascular Disease 1998.* Stationery Office, London.

Prineas RJ, Crow RS and Blackburn H (1982) *The Minnesota Code. Manual of electrocardiographic findings.* John Wright, Bristol.

Ramachandran A, Sathyamurthy I, Snehalatha C et al. (2001) Risk variables for coronary artery disease in Asian Indians. *Am J Cardiol.* **87**: 267–71.

Reaven GM (1988) Role of insulin resistance in human disease. *Diabetes.* **37**: 1595–607.

Ridker PM, Hennekens CH, Stampfer MJ, Manson JE and Vaughan DE (1994) Prospective study of endogenous tissue plasminogen activator and risk of stroke. *Lancet.* **343**: 940–3.

Rose GA and Blackburn H (1986) *Cardiovascular Survey Methods.* World Health Organization Monograph 56. WHO, Geneva.

Shah N, Heng CK, Mozoomdar BP et al. (1995) Racial variation of factor VII activity and antigen level and their correlates in healthy Chinese and Indians at low and high risk for coronary artery disease. *Atherosclerosis.* **117**: 33–42.

Shaukat N, de Bono DP and Jones DR (1995) Like father, like son? Sons of patients of European or Indian origin with coronary artery disease reflect their parents' risk factor pattern. *Br Heart J.* **74**: 318–23.

Shephard J, Blaugh GJ, Murphy MB et al. (2002) Pravastatin in elderly at risk of vascular disease (PROSPER): a randomized controlled trial. *Lancet.* **360**: 1623–30.

Thorn TJ (1989) International mortality from heart disease: rates and trends. *Int J Epidemiol.* **18**: S20–8.

WHO Expert Consultation (2004) Appropriate body-mass index for Asian population and its implications for policy and intervention strategies. *Lancet.* **363**: 157–63.

Wild S and McKeigue P (1997) Cross-sectional analysis of mortality by country of birth in England and Wales, 1970–92. *BMJ.* **314**: 705–10.

Wilhelmsen L, Svardsudd K, Korsan-Bengten K, Larsson B, Welin L and Tibblin G (1984) Fibrinogen as a risk factor for stroke and myocardial infarction. *N Engl J Med* **311**: 501–5.

Wilkinson P, Sayer J, Laji K et al. (1996) Comparison of case fatalities in south Asians and white patients after acute myocardial infarction: observational study. *BMJ.* **312**: 1330–3.

Chapter 8

Stroke and the Indo-Asians

Introduction

Stroke is a common condition and has major impact on the lives of sufferers and their carers. Each year 110 000 new strokes are diagnosed in England and Wales and a further 30 000 people have recurrence of their stroke. Within this cohort, 10 000 patients are aged under 55 years while 1000 are under 30 years of age. Stroke affects the elderly population and three-quarters of cases will be over the age of 65 and half will be over 75 years of age.

Worldwide, every year approximately 750 000 patients suffer from stroke with an annual mortality rate of 150 000.

In the UK, stroke is the third most common cause of death and 60 000 patients die each year. Approximately 30% of stroke patients die in the first month and most within the first 10 days. Of those who survive the first year, 65% will live independently and the rest will be significantly disabled; 5% will need to go into a residential or nursing home.

The economic burden of stroke is enormous. In 2002, expenditure on stroke care in the UK was £2.3 billion (5% of the total NHS budget). In 1991, 7.7 million working days were lost and the cost of lost production was around £445 million.

Worldwide, stroke is the third most common cause of death after heart disease and cancer and two-thirds of cases occur in developing countries. In 1990 3% of the world's burden for disability was caused by stroke and this is going to rise because of an increase in the elderly population in the developing world.

Definition

Transient ischaemic attack (TIA) is defined as 'a clinical syndrome characterised by an acute loss of focal cerebral or monocular function with symptoms lasting for less than 24 hours and which is thought to be due to inadequate cerebral or ocular blood supply as a result of low blood flow, arterial thrombosis or embolism associated with disease of the arteries, heart or blood'.

The definition of a stroke is 'a clinical syndrome characterised by rapidly developing clinical symptoms and/or signs of focal, and at times global (applied to patients in deep coma and those with subarachnoid haemorrhage), loss of cerebral function, with symptoms lasting more than 24 hours or leading to death, with no apparent cause other than that of vascular origin'.

Incidence and prevalence

The overall incidence of stroke is 2.4/1000 per annum in the developed countries with no comparable data from the developing world (Asia, Africa and

South America). The incidence of first stroke increases with age from 2/1000 per year in those aged 55–64 to 20/1000 per year in those aged 85+. It is, therefore, a disease of older people and three-quarters of all first strokes occur after the age of 65 years. The incidence of primary intracerebral haemorrhage may be higher in Asia and Africa than in the Western population.

The incidence of TIA is 0.42/1000 per year. The prevalence of stroke survivors is 5–7/1000. There are hardly any data on the incidence of stroke in the Indo-Asian population. Most of the evidence is collated from small studies carried out in the white, black and Chinese populations.

A study looking at ethnic differences in the incidence of first-ever stroke in south London found a crude annual incidence rate of 1.3 per 1000 population per year (Table 8.1). The total study population (234 533) included 72% whites, 21% blacks and 3% Indo-Asians ('Asians', Pakistanis, Bangladeshis); 612 patients with first strokes were registered in the community stroke register. The 'other' group included Asians, Indians, Pakistanis, Bangladeshis, Chinese and others. The number of first strokes in the 'other' group was 21 out of a total of 612 and the mean age was 66.9 years. The annual incidence was 0.61 per 1000 per year. This was significantly lower than the 'white' and 'black' groups.

Table 8.1 Annual incidence rates for the elderly group

Age	White			Black			Others – Asians, Pakistani, Indians, Bangladeshi, Chinese and other		
	No of cases	Popu-lation	Rate	No of cases	Popu-lation	Rate	No of cases	Popu-lation	Rate
65–74	139	15 192	4.57	34	1595	10.66	4	366	5.46
75–84	161	9410	8.55	12	358	16.76	4	166	12.05
>85	88	2454	17.93	5	39	64.10	3	43	34.88
Total (all ages)	469	167 834	1.46	102	49 499	1.03	21	17 200	0.61

Types and classification of stroke

Stroke occurs when there is a disturbance of blood supply to the brain. There are two main types of stroke (Table 8.2).

- *Ischaemic stroke*: this is the main cause of stroke and occurs in 80% of cases. This could be due to *in situ* thrombosis of lacunar or a major intracerebral blood vessel. The other cause could be a shower of embolic debri coming from the major blood vessels (carotid or vertebro-basilar arteries) or from the left chambers of the heart.
- *Haemorrhagic stroke*: this is due to rupture of a blood vessel and is seen in 20% of cases, of which primary intracerebral haemorrhage constitutes 15% and subarachnoid haemorrhage 5%.

Table 8.2 Classification of stroke and prognosis

	Lacunar (LACS)	Partial anterior circulation (PACS)	Total anterior circulation (TACS)	Posterior circulation (POCS)
Signs	Motor or sensory loss only	Two of: motor, sensory loss or cortical involvement: hemianopia	All of: motor, sensory loss or cortical involvement: hemianopia	Hemianopia, brain stem or cerebellar signs
Dead at 1 year (%)	10	20	60	20
Dependent at 1 year (%)	25	30	35	20

Causes of ischaemic stroke

There are more than 130 causes of stroke which can be grouped under the following headings.

- *Vascular* (75%): atherothrombo-embolic disease of extracranial and/or large intracranial arteries – 50%; occlusion of small deep lacunar arteries – 25%.
- *Cardio-embolism* (20%).
- *Miscellaneous*: (5%): haematological.

Vascular causes

- Atherothromboembolism: vascular embolic, occlusive thrombotic, low blood flow.
- Vasculitis: SLE, Giant cell arteritis, systemic necrotising vasculitis, Takayasu's, Kawasaki's disease, antiphospholipid syndrome, rheumatoid disease, etc.
- Arterial dissection: Marfan's & Ehlers–Danos syndrome, psudoxanthoma elasticum, fibromuscular dysplasia, trauma, cystic medial necrosis.

Cardio-embolic causes

- atrial fibrillation leading to thromboembolism
- infective endocarditis
- mural thrombus from recent myocardial infarction, cardiomyopathy, mechanical valves, calcium embolism from valves
- rheumatic endocarditis
- atrial myxoma
- paradoxical embolism through patent foramen ovale and atrial septal defect.

Haematological causes

- *Thrombophilia*: factor V Leiden-heterozygote, protein C and S and antithrombin III deficiency
- *Hyperviscosity syndromes*: polycythaemia, multiple myeloma
- *Immunological disorders*: antiphospholipid syndrome
- *Quantitative abnormalities*: leukaemia, essential thrombocythaemia
- *Qualitative abnormalities*: haemoglobinopathies: thalassaemia, sickle cell disease.

The approximate frequency of the main causes of stroke in the white population is:

- atherothromboembolism   50%
- intracranial small vessel disease   25%
- embolism from the heart   20%
- other causes   5%.

A stroke could have a single cause but usually there is a mixture of several causes.

Causes of cerebral haemorrhage

Changes in cerebral circulation:

- microaneurysm and lipohyalinosis of small penetrating vessels
- arterio-venous malformation
- amyliod angiopathy
- saccular aneurysm
- angioma
- venous thrombosis
- arterial dissection
- vasculitis.

Haemodynamic changes:

- arterial hypertension.

Haematological conditions:

- anticoagulants
- antiplatelets agents
- thrombolytics
- haemophilia
- thromocytopenia.

Other rare causes:

- bleeding into a intracerebral tumour

- alcohol
- cocaine
- amphetamine
- other sympathomimetics.

Risk factors

There are many risk factors influencing the chance of developing a stroke. Some of these risk factors and their associated relative risk are listed below (Table 8.3). The risk factors could be conventional or novel.

Conventional risk factors

Table 8.3 Conventional risk factors

Risk factors	Relative risk
Age (<64 v 75+)	5
Hypertension	7
Current smoking	4
Atrial fibrillation	3.5–6.9
Ischaemic heart disease	3
Heart failure	5
Past TIA	5.2
Diabetes mellitus	2.2
Acute alcohol intoxication	5 (men only)
Raised triglycerides (<6.5 mmol/L)	2.4
Low social class	1.6

TIA = transient ischaemic attack.

Other factors include male sex, obesity, sleep apnoea, polycythaemia, migraine, oestrogen therapy, climate and air quality. Several factors might come into play in the causation of a stroke.

Novel risk factors

Physiological prothrombotic factors could precipitate a stroke if they are stimulated by environmental effects. Extreme climatic conditions are sometimes responsible for stimulating these factors. Most novel risk factors seem to accelerate atherosclerosis.

Homocysteine level in plasma is a novel and independent risk factor in Indo-Asians. Raised levels of homocysteine concentration may be related to reduced intake of vitamins B12 and B6 and folic acid. A study has suggested that supplementing these vitamins in the diet may have some influence in reducing atherosclerosis.

Another study reported that lowering homocysteine levels by giving folic acid and vitamin B6 supplements to healthy siblings of patients with premature atherothrombotic disease favourably influenced the course of atherosclerosis.

Box 8.1 Novel risk factors

- Raised plasminogen activator inhibitor-1
- Raised lipoprotein (a)
- Raised homocysteine concentration
- Infections (*Helicobacter pylori*, *Chlamydia pneumoniae*)
- Genetic polymorphism
- Rheological markers (raised C-reactive protein, raised fibrinogen)

Pathogenesis

Stroke is believed to result from rupture of unstable atherosclerotic plaques, leading to the development of thrombosis and acute occlusion of a critical artery. This process is complex. As the causes of stroke are so varied, the pathogenesis is heterogeneous. The conventional vascular risk factors include increasing age, diabetes, hypertension, tobacco smoking and dyslipidaemia.

A Canadian study has shown that Indo-Asians subjects had a greater degree of atherosclerosis and plaque instability when compared with European and Chinese cohorts. This study measured the mean maximum intimal medial thickness (MM-IMT) of the carotid arteries using carotid B-mode ultrasonography. The European group had the greatest MM-IMT of 0.75 mm, the Chinese had the lowest (0.69 mm) while the Indo-Asians had an intermediate MM-IMT of 0.72 mm.

Attitude towards rehabilitation

Name of the condition

There are only a few special words to describe stroke syndrome in the Indian subcontinent. In the Eastern states of Punjab, it is sometimes called *ardh anga* (*ardh* = half, *anga* = body) while in the rest of the Indian subcontinent it is known as *lakuya*. In Pakistan the Urdu word for stroke is *falij*.

Attitudes and beliefs

Rehabilitation should start early in a stroke rehabilitation unit with the aim of restoring function and reducing the impact of stroke on the patients and their carers. Formal rehabilitation in a stroke unit will reduce death and disability and also reduce the length of stay in hospital.

The concept of physical rehabilitation is not widely understood by Indo-Asian elders. When someone is ill, they remain in bed until they improve or die. The belief that bed rest is essential to recuperate from an illness probably comes from experiences gathered from previous generations. Serious life-threatening infectious diseases like smallpox, typhoid, cholera and tuberculosis in the pre-antibiotic era demanded bed rest because of extreme debilitation and weakness. Therefore active rehabilitation may be thought to be unhelpful and unnecessary.

Major neurological illnesses occurring in the Indian subcontinent include poliomyelitis, leprosy, paraplegia due to spinal cord injury. These conditions lead to immense suffering through poverty and the patients usually end up begging for subsistence. This negative attitude towards these conditions may be reflected in stroke rehabilitation. The stroke teams must carefully explain the pathology and prognosis of the stroke. This is followed by skilful negotiation on the aims, goals and methods of rehabilitation with the patient and the family.

Personal and daily activities of daily living (PADL and DADL) are used in Western hospital settings to assess progress and discharge planning. These goals may not be reflected in the rehabilitation targets for Indo-Asians elders who have different customs of dressing, bathing, toileting, cooking and eating. These differences must be taken into account.

Many Indo-Asian elders believe in the benefits of massaging with vegetable oils like mustard oil or sesame seed oil. They might abandon their hospital therapy programme and return to their country of origin for herbal and massage treatment. This practice is common and will break the treatment regimen given by the physiotherapist. Again careful negotiation will be needed to achieve the treatment goals set with the patient and their carers.

Health beliefs

There are many beliefs that can determine how someone views the causation of illness like stroke. One belief might be that it is God who has caused the disease and prayers will help in its alleviation. Some might see the disease as a result of previous negative deeds (*karma*) and a feeling of resignation and inevitability will prevail. Traditional beliefs are that spirits or the 'evil eye' has caused the illness, particularly a stroke, and this must be dealt with quasi-religious or para-normal rituals. Patients might return to their villages of their country of origin and employ witch doctors to perform these rituals. The Western-trained medical professional might see these beliefs as irrational and illogical.

Social factors

When planning transfer to the primary care setting, several things must be considered. Indo-Asian elders are at risk because they:

- are old
- suffer from cultural and racial discrimination
- have poor access to healthcare, housing, voluntary and social services
- have poor income and may live in abject poverty
- have to cope with the language barrier.

Management

Stroke unit care

Stroke unit care is associated with the long-term reduction of mortality (odds ratio (OR) 0.83; 95% confidence interval (CI) 0.69–0.98). There is also a reduction in the combined poor outcome of death or dependency (OR 0.69; 95% CI 0.59–0.82) and death or institutionalisation (OR 0.75; 95% CI 0.65–0.87).

Patients with suspected stroke therefore should be admitted and managed in a stroke unit as early as possible. This facility should be resourced to cater for the acute and rehabilitation aspects of stroke care.

Any patient with moderate or severe symptoms should be referred to hospital with the expectation of admission to a stroke unit.

Acute medical treatment

Aspirin

Aspirin should be started as soon as possible after the onset of symptoms if the diagnosis of cerebral haemorrhage is excluded by a CT or MR scan. The dose of aspirin is 150–300 mg a day given orally (rectally or intravenously if the patient is unable to swallow) to reduce morbidity and mortality, usually for two weeks. Thereafter 75–150 mg a day is sufficient. When aspirin is commenced within the first 48 hours after an ischaemic, stroke death and dependency is reduced at six months' follow up (relative risk reduction: 3%). Anticoagulation does not lead to overall benefit when given in ischaemic stroke. Early anticoagulation is indicated when there is a very high risk of embolism.

Heparin

Heparin, low molecular weight heparins or heparinoids lower the risk of arterial and venous thromboembolism but the risk of haemorrhage offsets the benefits. Patients who are at high risk of deep vein thrombosis should be prescribed compression stockings or prophylactic low molecular weight heparin.

Thrombolysis

Thrombolysis with tissue plasminogen activator (tPA; alteplase 0.9 mg/kg over one hour) should only be given in ischaemic stroke within three hours of onset of symptoms. It increases survival and reduces disability but can cause fatal intracerebral haemorrhage in about 5% of patients. Alteplase is licensed in the USA, Canada and some European countries, including the UK where its use is restricted to certain centres.

Secondary prevention of stroke and other vascular risk factors

Hypertension should not be lowered in acute stroke patients, particularly in the first week, unless there is accelerated hypertension or symptoms and signs of aortic dissection.

Hyperglycaemia should be maintained within normal range, if necessary with insulin.

- Aspirin should be given as soon as possible after the onset of stroke if a diagnosis of haemorrhage is considered unlikely. Aspirin dose: 150–300 mg a day.
- Anticoagulation should be considered in all patients with atrial fibrillation and started 14 days after onset of stroke provided intracerebral haemorrhage has been excluded.
- Thrombolysis with alteplase should only be administered within three hours of onset of ischaemic stroke and only if cerebral haemorrhage has been excluded.
- Blood pressure should not be lowered in the first week unless there is accelerated hypertension or aortic dissection. Existing antihypertensive medications should be continued.
- Blood sugar should be maintained within normal range.
- Hydration should be maintained within normality.
- Pyrexia should be controlled.

Brain imaging

A CT scan or MRI is essential in the classification of stroke pathology and identifying stroke mimics, e.g. tumours, subdural haematoma. MR arteriogram and, rarely, cerebral angiogram could be done to delineate intracerebral arteries. Extracranial arteries are assessed by carotid duplex scan or CT angiogram. MR venograms are done to delineate the cortical veins.

Brain imaging (CT or MRI) should be done on all patients to detect intracerebral or subarachnoid haemorrhage and exclude other causes of stroke, within 48 hours of onset.
Urgent brain scans are indicated when there is:

- depressed level of consciousness
- papilloedema, neck stiffness or fever
- unexplained, progressive or fluctuating symptoms
- severe headache at onset
- indication for thrombolysis or early anticoagulation
- history of anticoagulant therapy or known bleeding diathesis
- history of head injury prior to onset of symptoms.

MRI should be considered if CT scan is normal and the diagnosis of stroke is in doubt. This is especially indicated in patients with brain stem or cerebellar symptoms or to exclude old cerebral haemorrhage.
Patients with carotid TIA should be considered for brain imaging to exclude AV malformation, tumour or subdural haematoma.

For further details please consult the *National Clinical Guidelines for Stroke*, second edition, June 2004. The Royal College of Physians, 11 St Andrews Place, London, NW1 4LE. www.rcplondon.ac.uk

Driving and stroke

The Road Traffic Act of 1988 covers legal fitness to drive an automobile either a four- or a two-wheeler. Section 92 covers the physical disabilities of drivers. The Motor Vehicles (Driving Licences) Regulations 1996 is a further addendum to the driving laws. The DVLA will decide if a driver is medically fit to drive and has the legal responsibility to authorise this. For further information please consult the DVLA website.

Secondary prevention of stroke

Stroke survivors not only expect to regain complete independence but also would like to be protected from recurrence. The risk of recurrence is 7% per annum and about 30–40% over the first five years (Table 8.4).

There is evidence of effectiveness of secondary prevention and this is updated constantly. Such evidence is available for antihypertensive therapy, angiotensin-converting enzyme inhibition (ACEI) and angiotensin II receptor antagonists, antiplatelet therapy and carotid endarterectomy. There is evidence for stroke secondary prevention when smoking cessation can be achieved. Lipid-lowering drugs and anticoagulation strategies also contributes towards this goal.

Table 8.4 Risk reduction with various treatment strategies for TIAs and ischaemic stroke

Strategy	Stroke risk/year		Relative risk of recurrence (RRR) (95% CI)	Absolute risk reduction (ARR)	Number needed to treat (NNT)
	Control	Intervention			
Antihypertensive therapy	7%	5%	28% (17–38%)	2%	50
ACE inhibition	7%	5.5%	22% (14–30%)	1.5%	65
Aspirin	7%	6%	14% (4–21%)	1%	100
Clopidogrel	7%	5.4%	10% (3–17%)	1.6%	62
Dipyridamole + aspirin	7%	4.6%	23% (7–37%)	2.4%	42
Carotid endarterectomy	8.8%	4.6%	48% (22–73%)	2%	24
Lipid-lowering drugs	7%	5.3%	25% (8–38%)	1.7%	59
Smoking cessation	7%	4.7%	33% (29–38%)	2.3%	43

Blood pressure reduction

About 50% of ischaemic strokes are caused by atherothromboembolism and half of these patients have a history of hypertension. Following a TIA or a stroke, further lowering of blood pressure by 9/4 mmHg will reduce the relative risk of recurrence (RRR) of stroke by 28% and lowering blood pressure by 12/5 mmHg will reduce it by 43%. The absolute risk reduction (ARR) is 2%. Therefore the number of stroke patients who need to be treated (NNT) to prevent one stroke per annum is 50.

Diuretic therapy remains the most cost-effective option in the initiation of treatment for hypertension. The current annual cost for bendrofluazide is £10–15.

Angiotensin-converting enzyme inhibition

The Heart Outcome Prevention Evaluation (HOPE) trial studied 9297 symptomatic patients with a history of coronary, cerebral, peripheral vascular disease or diabetes mellitus, and randomised them to either ramipril 10 mg daily or placebo. There was a significant reduction in subsequent stroke, myocardial infarction or death due to any vascular cause (ramipril group 14% versus placebo 17.8%). The RRR and the ARR were 22% and 1.5% respectively per annum. The NNT was 65. The BP reduction was only 3/1 mmHg in the ramipril group, which supports the hypothesis that anti-atherogenic mechanisms may be operating.

Box 8.5 Hypertension

All patients should have their blood pressure checked and hypertension persisting for over one month treated according to the British Hypertension Society guidelines.

- Optimal treatment target   <140/<85 mmHg
- Minimum accepted level   <150/<90 mmHg
- Patients with diabetes   <130/<85 mmHg

Further reduction of blood pressure should be considered using a combination of long-acting ACE inhibitor (e.g. perindopril or ramipril) and a thiazide (e.g. indapamide).

Antiplatelet therapy

Aspirin

Low-dose sspirin reduces the RRR of stroke and TIAs by 14% and the ARR by 1%. The NNT is 100.

Aspirin and dipyridamole

When compared with aspirin, the combination of aspirin and dipyridamole (modified release) given twice a day reduces the RRR of stroke and TIAs by 23% and the ARR by 2.4%. The NNT is 42.

Clopidogrel

Clopidogrel, when compared with aspirin, reduces the RRR of all vascular events, including stroke and TIAs, by 10% and the ARR by 1.6%. The NNT is 62.

Box 8.6 Antiplatelet agents

All patients with ischaemic stroke who are not on anticoagulants should take antiplatelet agents.

- Aspirin 75–325 mg a day or
- Clopidogrel 75 mg a day or
- A combination of aspirin 25 mg and dipyridamole modified release 200 mg twice a day.

Aspirin-intolerant patients should be taking:

- Clopidogrel 75 mg a day or
- Dipyridamole modified release 200 mg twice a day.

Lipid-lowering drugs

The evidence linking hyperlipidaemia and coronary artery disease is strong. There is evidence that patients with stroke and hypercholesterolaemia and even normal cholesterol, when treated with a 3-hydroxy-3-methylglutaryl coenzyme A inhibitor (HGM CoA), popularly known as a statin, will reduce their RRR by 25% and their ARR by 1.7%. The NNT is 59.

Box 8.7 Lipid-lowering agents

A statin should be considered for all patients with a history of ischaemic heart disease and a cholesterol of <3.5 mmol/L following a stroke.

Carotid endarterectomy in symptomatic carotid stenosis

Carotid endarterectomy is indicated in patients with carotid territory stroke or TIAs who have severe stenosis (>70%) of the symptomatic artery. The patient must be fit and give informed consent. The operation reduces the relative risk by 48% and the ARR by 2.4%. The NNT is 24. The cost of the procedure and the perioperative morbidity have to be taken into account.

Box 8.8 Carotid endarterectomy in symptomatic carotid stenosis

Any patient with a carotid artery area stroke and minor or absent residual disability, or where carotid stenosis is measured at >70%, should be considered for carotid endarterectomy.

Table 8.5 Cardio-embolic TIA/ischaemic stroke due to atrial fibrillation

Strategy	Stroke rate/year		RRR	ARR	NNT
	Control	Intervention	(95% CI)		
Anticoagulation	12%	4%	67% (43–80%)	8%	12
Aspirin	12%	10%	14% (15–36%)	2%	50

Anticoagulation therapy

It is essential to prevent cardiac embolism by giving an anticoagulant. Warfarin sodium, phenindione and acenocoumarol (formerly called nicoumalone) are the drugs used. The target International Normalised Ratio (INR) of 2.0–3.0 should be aimed for when long-term therapy is indicated, particularly in atrial fibrillation (AF). Anticoagulation of patients with stroke or TIAs in AF reduces the RRR of stroke by 67% and the ARR by 8%. The NNT is 12.

Box 8.9 Anticoagulation

- Should be started in every patient with ischaemic stroke and AF (valvular or non-valvular) unless contraindicated.
- Should be considered for all patients with ischaemic stroke with mitral valve disease, prosthetic valves or within three months of myocardial infarction.
- Should **not** be used after TIAs or minor strokes unless cardiac embolism is suspected.
- Should **not** be started until brain imaging has excluded haemorrhage.
- Should be started after 14 days have passed from the onset of an ischaemic stroke where indicated.

Further reading

Anand SS, Yousef S, Vaksan V et al. (2000) Differences in risk factors, athero-sclerosis, and cardiovascular disease between ethnic groups in Canada: the

Study of Health Assessment and Risk in Ethnic groups (SHARE). *Lancet*. **356**: 279–84.

Bath PMW and Lees KR (2000) Acute stroke. *BMJ*. **320**: 920–3.

Chambers JC, Obeid OA, Refsum H et al. (2000) Plasma homocysteine concentration and risk of coronary heart disease in UK Indian, Asian and European men. *Lancet*. **335**: 523–7.

Department of Health (2001) *National Service Framework for Older People*. Department of Health, London.

DVLA (2001) *At a Glance Guide to the Current Medical Standards of Fitness to Drive*. DVLA, Swansea.

Ebrahim S (1990) *Clinical Epidemiology of Stroke*. Oxford University Press, Oxford.

Ebrahim S (1996) Ethnic elders. *BMJ*. **313**: 610–13.

Hankey GJ (2001) Secondary prevention of stroke and its cost-effectiveness. *Stroke Review*. **5**(4): 1–5.

Royal College of Physicians (2004) *National Clinical Guidelines for Stroke*. Royal College of Physicians, London.

Stewart JA, Dundas R, Howard RS et al. (1999) Ethnic differences in incidence of stroke: prospective study with stroke register. *BMJ* **318**: 967–71.

Stroke Unit Triallists' Collaboration (1997) Collaborative systematic review of the randomised trials of organised inpatients (stroke unit) care after stroke. *BMJ*. **314**: 1157–9.

Vermeulen EGJ, Stehouwer CDA, Twisk JWR et al. (2000) Effect of homocysteine-lowering treatment with folic acid plus vitamin B6 on progression of sub clinical atherosclerosis: a randomised, placebo-controlled trial. *Lancet*. **355**: 517–21.

Warlow CP, Dennis MS, van Gijn J et al. (eds) (2001) *Stroke: a practical guide to management* (2e). Blackwell Science, Oxford.

Chapter 9

Travellers' illnesses in Indo-Asian elders

Who are the travellers?

The Indian subcontinent is the ancestral home for most Indo-Asians and visiting at least once in their lifetime is essential. The Indo-Asians who arrived in the UK in the 1950s and 1960s have retired or are preparing to retire. Most Indo-Asian elders would like to visit the Indian subcontinent in the winter months and return to the UK in the spring to enjoy the British summer. The primary migrants will visit the towns or villages in the subcontinent where they originally came from. Secondary migrants will visit their countries of origin such as East Africa or the West Indies and also travel to the subcontinent. Many Hindu and Sikh emigrants will make pilgrimage to India whereas Muslim pilgrims will be going to Saudi Arabia for the *Hajj* or *Umra*. Many Shia Muslims will make trips to Iran and the Middle East to visit other holy sites.

Table 9.1 List of primary migrants to the UK

Country of origin	Main religious groups	Main states/areas of origin
Pakistan	Muslim	Mirpur, Azad Khasmir
Bangladesh	Muslim	Sylhet
India	Hindus	Punjab, Haryana, Gujrat, Bengal, Tamil Nadu
	Sikhs	Punjab
	Muslims	Northern states
	Christians	
Sri Lanka	Buddhists, Hindus	Colombo, Jafna
Nepal	Hindu	Kathmandu

Table 9.2 List of secondary migrants to the UK

Country/Region of origin	Main religious groups	Main states/ areas of origin
East Africa	Hindus, Sikhs	Uganda, Kenya, Malawi
West Indies	Hindus, Muslims, Christians	Caribbean islands
South East Asia Malaysia	Hindus, Sikhs	Singapore, Hong Kong,
Fiji	Hindus, Christians	Fijian islands

What attracts them to the Indian subcontinent?

The migrants' 'pull' to the Indian subcontinent is multifactorial. Indo-Asian elders wish to return to their birthplace and their ancestral homes during their lifetime and some wish to be buried there. In 1999 half a million people visited the Indian subcontinent.

This 'pull' has many aspects.

- Visiting family and friends.
- Attending family functions, e.g. weddings and funerals.
- Accompanying second-generation family to visit ancestral homes, villages or towns and making them aware of their family way of life.
- Looking after ancestral properties, e.g. family farm, houses, etc.
- Cultural visits, e.g. classical music and poetry events.
- Religious pilgrimages, e.g. some Hindu pilgrimage sites (Kedar Nath, Badri Nath and Gongtri) are in the Himalayas, so visitors may suffer altitude sickness and exacerbation of pre-existing cardiac conditions. Travel in the desert (Pushar) may aggravate pre-existing renal failure or cause heat exhaustion or heat stroke. Muslims going to Saudi Arabia for the *Hajj* may be exposed to similar problems.
- Sight-seeing and discovering the subcontinent.
- Business travellers.
- Conferences and professional meetings.
- Trying traditional medical therapy, e.g. Ayurvedic medicine, massage treatment in stroke and occasionally regular treatment like cataract extraction.

Getting medical treatment in the Indian subcontinent

Many elders from the Indian subcontinent who visit their families may get medical and surgical treatment while they are there. They use the system to jump the National Health Service waiting list for conditions like cataract extraction, joint surgery, coronary artery bypass graft, angioplasty and, rarely, renal transplant which is acquired illegally. Other attractions for using the local health services include privileges of cheap private healthcare and recuperation with relatives. The quality of surgical facilities is excellent in metropolitan cities but can be questionable in provincial towns. Blood transfusion can be dangerous if the blood is acquired from unscrupulous sources. Serious blood-borne conditions such as AIDS, hepatitis and malaria can be acquired. These points need to be borne in mind when dealing with a patient who has received medical treatment abroad.

Preparations for travel

Falling ill in the tropics, due to a disease or an injury, is not unusual and can be prevented by educating and immunising the traveller and supplying them with medical equipment. The health risks of international travel are very high. Of the 1 000 000 travellers who will visit the developing countries and stay for a month, half (500 000) will develop some sort of health problem, 8000 will have to see a physician, 300 will have to be hospitalised but only one will die.

The common non-serious illnesses the traveller will face are diarrhoea, upper respiratory tract infection and skin sepsis due to insect bite. Serious illnesses, and occasionally death, may occur from road traffic accidents, exacerbation of chronic illness (e.g. ischaemic heart disease, heart failure, diabetes, renal failure) and drowning. The health risks will depend on the conditions of travel, such as staying with family or friends, in a five-star hotel or backpacking, age of traveller and area visited.

Pre-travel health assessment

Assessment of the traveller's current health status must be made, including chronic illnesses like epilepsy, diabetes, heart disease, blood dyscrasia and psychological illnesses. Allergies to drugs, food, particularly eggs, and the environment will have an impact on the choice of immunisation and chemoprophylaxis.

Review of travel itinerary

- Dates of travel, including season. The monsoon season will make travellers more prone to mosquito-borne diseases and diarrhoeal illnesses.
- Type of accommodation: air-conditioned accommodation reduces the risk of mosquito bites.
- Type of travel: road traffic accidents are common.
- Places to be visited: high-altitude destinations can cause altitude sickness.

Recommended immunisation for Indo-Asian elders

Table 9.3 Routine immunisation for Indo-Asian elders

Vaccine	Comments
Tetanus/diphtheria	Worldwide
Poliomyelitis	Live oral vaccine
Influenza	
Pneumococcal	>65 years, pulmonary disease, duration 5 years

Table 9.4 Recommended immunisation

Vaccine	Comments
Hepatitis A	2–4 weeks before departure, second dose confers 10+ years' immunity
Hepatitis B	As above
Typhoid	Parenteral or live oral vaccine
Rabies	2 years' protection
Japanese encephalitis	Duration 3 years. Outbreaks in Kathmandu valley in Nepal

Table 9.5 Required or essential immunisation

Vaccine	Comments
Yellow fever	Live vaccine. International certificate of vaccination essential. Give 10 days before arrival. Needed for travel to Africa
Meningococcal meningitis	Essential to visit Saudi Arabia, particularly for *Hajj* pilgrims. Give 10 days before arrival

Cholera immunisation, oral or parenteral, is not recommended.

For Muslim pilgrims going for the *Hajj*, there are strict immunisation guidelines issued by the Saudi government.

Travel advice

- *Travellers' diarrhoea:* this will affect 30–60% of travellers within two weeks of travel and usually lasts for four days. Contaminated food rather than water is the usual cause. Do not consume ice and salads. Before buying bottled water, always check the cap is intact. Personal water filters are effective. Self-treatment of diarrhoea should include aggressive hydration with salt and sugar solution, plus antimotility agents. Ciprofloxacin is a popular self-medication though resistance to it is increasing.
- *Insect-borne diseases:* insects are attracted to humans by their body odour and the emission of carbon dioxide and lactic acid. Mosquitos tend to bite more at dusk. Houseflies and cockroaches carry enterotoxic bacteria and viruses so covering non-refrigerated food with netting is crucial. Travellers are advised to wear light-coloured, loose-fitting garments covering their limbs, use insect repellents and spray bed nets and clothing with insecticide (permethrin or deltamethrin). Mosquito coils may reduce exposure.
- *Environmental risks:* travellers who swim or bathe in ponds and rivers in religious sites are prone to water-borne diseases like leptospirosis, giardia, hepatitis A and Norwalk virus infections. Walking barefoot may cause cutaneous larva migrans from hookworm and *Stronglyloides stercoralis* larvae.
- *Heat or cold exposure:* sunburn, heat exhaustion and heat stroke are common if precautions are not taken. Use of sun cream (at least SPF 10), adequate hydration and salt intake is crucial in the process of recovery. Hypothermia and altitude sickness can occur when visiting religious pilgrimage sites in the Himalayas. Altitude sickness usually occurs above 2500 metres above sea level. Patients with cardiovascular disease are particularly prone to worsening of their symptoms at high altitude due to low oxygen tension.
- *Trauma:* injury is the greatest unforeseen danger to the traveller. Fractures of bones and serious internal injuries can occur following a road traffic accident, falls and swimming. Travellers are more prone (4–5 times) to road traffic accidents than local people as they are not aware of the local traffic etiquettes. Seatbelt laws are just being introduced in the Indian subcontinent. Older vehicles and coaches will not have seatbelts and the culture of wearing them does not exist. Travellers who are not immunised must get tetanus immunisation. Cellulitis and wound infections will need active treatment.

- *Bites and stings:* animal bites can cause rabies and make the wound turn septic if adequate precautions are not taken. Dogs and bats are the usual vectors of rabies. Worldwide, approximately 50 000 cases of rabies are reported every year. Bites from reptiles (cobras), arachnids (spiders and scorpions) and insects (bees, wasps) can be fatal.
- *Ingestion:* Consuming illicit drinks as part of a religious experience can cause hallucinations, optic nerve damage, liver failure and death. Contaminated food and water will cause a multitude of illnesses, described later in the chapter.

Incubation periods

Table 9.6 Short incubation period of less than 10 days

Illness	Organisms	Incubation period	Mode of transmission	Vector	Comments
Enteric fever	*Salmonella typhi, paratyphi A, B, C*	Less than 1 week	Faeco–oral	Human to human	Undercooked and raw food Can be fatal
Enteric viral infections	Hepatitis A, Norwalk, adenovirus, rotavirus, enterovirus, calciviruses, astroviruses	Less than 1 week	Faeco–oral	Human to human	Self-limiting
Enteric bacterial infections	*Salmonella, Shigella, Campylobacter, E. coli*			Human to human	Poor sanitation
Dengue, dengue haemorrhagic fever	Arbovirus	3–15 days (usually 5–8 days)	Inoculation	Mosquito, *Aedes aegypti*	Debilitating. Can be fatal
Japanese encephalitis	Arbovirus				Can be fatal
Rabies	Rabies virus	7 days to several years (70% less than 60 days)	Saliva of infected animals	Canids (dogs, fox) bats, cats, other farm animals	Causes encephalomyelitis. Can be fatal
Tetanus	*Clostridium tetani*	5 days to 15 weeks (average 8–12 days)	Wound contamination	Spores of the organism in the soil	Can be fatal

Table 9.7 Medium incubation period of 11–21 days

Illness	Organisms	Incubation period	Mode of transmission	Vector	Comments
Malaria	*Plasmodium falciparum*	7–30 days	Inoculation	Mosquito bite female *Anopheles*	Falciparum infection can be fatal
Typhoid	Salmonella *enterica serovar typhi, serovar paratyphi* A, B & C	Less than a week to 3 weeks	Faeco–oral	Human to human	Food and water contaminated with faeces
Hepatitis A Leptospirosis			Faeco–oral Skin contact	Urine of rodents	Fresh water pools or rivers
Amoebiasis	*Entamoeba histolytica*		Faeco–oral	Human to human	Contaminated food and water. Cysts destroyed by boiling and filtration
Visceral larva migrans	*Toxocara canis, T. cati*	A few days to several months	Faeco–oral	Dog or cat hookworm ingestion	Walking barefoot
Cholera	*Vibrio cholerae O1* (classic & El-Tor) & O139 (Bengal)	1–5 days	Faeco–oral	Human to human	Water-borne
Giardiasis	*Giardia lamblia*	A few weeks to several months	Faeco–oral	Human to human	Contaminated food and water

Table 9.8 Long incubation period of more than 30 days

Illness	Organisms	Incubation period	Mode of transmission	Vector	Comments
Malaria	*Plasmodium vivax, ovale* and *malariae*	3–6 months, may take longer	Inoculation	Mosquito bite female *Anopheles*	
Tuberculosis					
Visceral leishmaniasis	*Leishmania donovani*	2–8 months	Inoculation	Sand flies	North-east India and Bangladesh
Filariasis	*Wuchereria bancrofti, Brugia malayi*	Many months after first exposure	Inoculation	Mosquito species *Anopheles, Culex* and *Aedes, Mansonia*	

Table 9.8 Long incubation period of more than 30 days (*continued*)

Illness	Organisms period	Incubation transmission	Mode of	Vector	Comments
Amoebic liver abscess	*Entamoeba histolytica*				
Helminthic infections	*Ascaris lumbricoides, Ankylostoma*		Faeco–oral, inoculation	Dog, pig, cattle	
Hepatitis B, C			Blood-borne	Human to human	Infected needles, sexual

Descriptions of symptoms and illnesses

Pyrexia

Fever is a serious presentation of illness in the returned traveller. The most important causes are malaria, enteric fever, septicaemia, hepatitis, amoebic liver abscess, respiratory tract infections and arbovirus infections.

Pyrexia may be acute (<14 days) or chronic (>14 days).

Box 9.1 Types of fevers

Fevers with anaemia
Malaria
Sickle cell, thalassaemia,
G6PD deficiency

Relapsing fevers
Malaria
Visceral leishmaniasis
Filariasis
Cholangitis
Borrelia

Life-threatening fevers
Malaria
Typhoid
Dengue haemorrhagic fever

Fever with leucocytosis
Deep abscess
Amoebic liver abscess
Cholangitis
Relapsing fever

Fever with eosinophilia
Microfilaria
Visceral larva migrans

Fever with neutropenia
Malaria
Disseminated TB
Visceral leishmaniasis
Brucellosis
HIV infection

Malaria

There are four species of malaria, of which *Plasmodium vivax* is the most common and *P. falciparum* the most dangerous. The risk of catching malaria is high when visiting the Indian subcontinent and this includes the large cities. The disease is more severe in the elderly.

Drug-resistant strains of *Plasmodium* are noted throughout the world. *P. falciparum* is resistant to chloroquine and mefloquine while *P. vivax* is resistant to chloroquine.

The majority of travellers who contract malaria will exhibit the symptoms when they return home. The latent periods are shown in Box 9.2.

Box 9.2 Latent periods of malarial strains

P. falciparum 7–60 days
P. vivax 90–180 days
P. ovale 90 days–1 year
P. malariae 90 days–1 year

Chemoprophylaxis

Complete 100% protection is never achieved with malaria chemoprophylaxis. The main aim is to prevent deaths from falciparum malaria. Travellers who do not take chemoprophylaxis and visit the Indian subcontinent for one month or more have a malaria risk of 1:250. Currently there is no vaccine available for malaria prevention. Many travellers abandon their medications because of ignorance, adverse side effects and misinformation they have heard or read in the media. Some even resort to homeopathy or traditional (Aurovedic) medicine.

Chemoprophylactic drugs are recommended for travellers visiting the Indian subcontinent and will depend on the regions visited. The relative risks of infectivity are noted below.

Variable risk

Table 9.9 Variable risk of acquiring malaria

	Pakistan	Sri Lanka	India	Bangladesh	Nepal
Risk variable and chloroquine resistance	Risk below 2000 metres	No risk in Colombo and south of it	+ (no risk in the mountain states)	+ (except Chittagong Hills)	Below 1300 metres, (in Kathmandu)

Treatment consists of chloroquine 300 mg once a week plus proguanil (Paludrine®) 200 mg daily.

High risk

Table 9.10 **High risk of acquiring malaria**

	Pakistan	Sri Lanka	India	Bangladesh	Nepal
Chloroquine resistance high				Only in Chittagong Hill Tracts	

Treatment consists of mefloquine (Lariam®) 250 mg once a week or doxy-cycline 100 mg once a day or Malarone® (proguanil 100 mg + atovaquone 250 mg) one tablet daily.

Duration of chemoprophylaxis
Start at least one week before travel and continue for four weeks after return except with Malarone®, which can be stopped one week after leaving an endemic area.

Table 9.11 **Reported cases of malaria in UK in the last 10 years**

Total reported cases	Deaths
21 919	104

Enteric fever

Enteric fever is transmitted from contaminated raw food, especially salads, undercooked food, including shellfish, water and ice. *Salmonella typhi* and *S. paratyphi* are the causative organisms. Fever increases in a stepwise fashion and is associated with headache, abdominal pain, diarrhoea or constipation and cough. Blood, stool and urine cultures help in confirming the diagnosis. The Widal test can be insensitive. Self-prescribing of antibiotics like ciprofloxacin will reduces the sensitivity of the laboratory tests. Case fatality rate from typhoid is 1.5%. Immunisation is available.

Dengue

Dengue is caused by arboviruses. There are four serotypes which are transmitted by *Aedes aegypti* mosquitoes. Fever, chills and rigours, severe myalgia, arthralgia ('break-bone' fever) and retro-orbital headache are some of the typical clinical features.

Dengue haemorrhagic fever and dengue shock syndrome are life-threatening conditions and are associated with bleeding diathesis, thrombocytopenia, haemoconcentration, hypoalbuminaemia, hypotension and shock.

Box 9.3 WHO grading of dengue haemorrhagic fever

I   Positive tourniquet test and/or easy bruising
II   Spontaneous bleeding
III Early signs of circulatory failure
IV Profound shock

Leptospirosis

Leptospirosis is caused by a spirochaete, *Leptosira haemorrhagica*. Fresh water is contaminated with urine of infected animals (particularly rats). The traveller contracts the disease by bathing, swimming or wading in ponds, lakes, lagoons or rivers, which could be part of a religious experience, or drinking contaminated water. Fever, chills, nausea and vomiting, myalgia and conjunctival suffusion may ensue. A second phase develops in 5–10% of cases (Weil's disease) and causes renal failure, jaundice, meningitis, adult respiratory distress syndrome and pulmonary haemorrhage.

Diarrhoea

Travellers going to the Indian subcontinent are at high risk (>20%) of developing acute diarrhoea. Half of all travellers on a two-week trip will get acute diarrhoea. Acute diarrhoea is defined as having three or more watery stools in 24 hours.

Table 9.12 Organisms causing acute diarrhoea

Classification	Organisms
Viral	Hepatitis A, Norwalk, rotavirus, adenovirus, calicivirus, astrovirus
Bacteria	*Escherichia coli, Campylobacter jejuni, Salmonella* species, *Shigella* species, *Bacillus cereus, Vibrio parahaemolyticus, V. cholerae, Staphylococcus aureus, Clostridia, Legionella pneumophilia*
Toxins	*Clostridium difficile*, fish, shellfish
Parasites	Malaria

Chronic diarrhoea occurs in a small number of travellers returning from the Indian subcontinent. About a quarter will complain of diarrhoea lasting for more than three weeks and 3% for more than four weeks.

Table 9.13 Organisms causing chronic diarrhoea

Classification	Organisms
Parasites	*Giardia, Entamoeba histolytica, Cryptosporidium* species, *Cyclospora* species
Helminths	*Ascaris lumbricoides, Strongyloides* species
Bacteria	*Camplylobacter jejuni, Yersinia* species, *E. coli*

Special features of travellers' diarrhoea

- *Campylobacter* infection can trigger Guillain–Barré syndrome.
- *Shigella* diarrhoea can induce Reiter's syndrome.
- *Yersinia* infection can mimic acute appendicitis.
- Diarrhoea can be a presenting feature of malaria.
- Prolonged doxycycline chemoprophylaxis for malaria can cause *Clostridium difficile* pseudomembranous enterocolitis.
- *Cryptosporidium* species can cause fatal diarrhoea in immune-compromised patients.
- Malabsorption can be due to parasitic and helminthic infections.
- Diarrhoea can derange drug absorption, e.g. chemoprophylaxis for malaria, antiepileptics, anti-diabetic medications, anticoagulants, etc.

Respiratory tract infections

Respiratory infections, particularly upper respiratory infections (URTI), are very common. Air pollution will aggravate or induce URTI. The usual organisms are viral URTI, viral (influenza, SARS) and bacterial pneumonia. Legionnaire's disease is associated with travel. Primary tuberculosis and Leoffler's syndrome are uncommon but should be considered in anyone returning from the Indian subcontinent.

Assessment of travellers returning from the Indian subcontinent

- Detailed pre-morbid and travel history, including areas of the countries visited. Duration and conditions of stay, details of and compliance with chemoprophylaxis and immunisations.
- Physical examination, particularly looking for fever, jaundice, signs of weight loss, lymphadenopathy, hepatosplenomegaly, chest and neurological signs. The character and consistency of diarrhoea should be noted.

Table 9.14 Investigations required for determining the cause of an infection

Investigations	Comments
Full blood count	Leucocytosis: bacterial infections Leucopenia: typhoid, overwhelming infections, viral Eosinophilia: Leoffler's syndrome
Blood film for malaria	
Liver function tests	Hepatitis, Weil's disease
Urea and electrolytes	Dehydration, renal function assessment
Culture	Urine: UTI, typhoid Stool: culture Sputum: pneumonia, TB Blood: typhoid, septicaemia CSF: meningococcal meningitis Bone marrow: TB, typhoid
Stool microscopy	Ova, cysts
Serology	Amoebiasis, arbovirus, typhoid, *C. difficile*, Lyme disease, hepatitis, parasites
Skin tests	TB
Biopsy	Bone marrow: TB, typhoid, leishmaniasis
Radiology	Chest: pneumonia, TB
	Ultrasonography: liver abscess, cysts
	CT/MRI: cystocercosis tuberculoma
Sigmoidoscopy	Colitis

Further reading

Davidson RN, Pasvol G (2001) Tropical infections Parts 1 and 2. *Medicine.* **29:5**; **29:6**. Medicine International Ltd.

Spira AM (2003) Assessment of travellers who return home ill. *Lancet.* **361**: 1459–69.

Spira AM (2003) Preparing the traveller. *Lancet.* **361**: 1368–81.

WHO (1997) *Dengue Haemorrhagic Fever: diagnosis, treatment, prevention and control* (2e). WHO, Geneva.

WHO (2000) Severe falciparum malaria. *Trans Roy Soc Trop Med Hyg*; **94** (Suppl. 1).

Chapter 10

Psychiatric problems in Indo-Asians

Social and cultural influences

Social and cultural influences are the most important factors in shaping an individual's personality. Culture could affect psychological behaviour in many ways but, on the other hand, psychiatric illness could be an effect of a culture. In other words, culture can influence the presentation of psychiatric illness.

Symptoms which may seem bizarre to a health professional trained in the West would be perfectly understandable with insight into the cultural life of Indo-Asian communities. Entities which fall within the textbook descriptions of Western psychiatry may be acceptable to certain ethnic groups. The background of the Indo-Asian community in the UK varies widely but there is broad agreement upon most areas of normality.

The main issue to be considered before discussing the pathology of psychiatric abnormalities in Indo-Asian communities is the limits of normality. For decades, cultural anthropologists have debated the definition of normality and abnormality in various cultures. Social definitions of normality and abnormality are based upon shared beliefs within a community. These boundaries could be loosely applied in certain areas but may be well defined in others. These social laws are unlikely to be written down, as is the case for criminal and corporate law. Some social norms are more fluid and change within a short time frame but others are rigidly embedded in the structure of the community and may not change even after centuries.

Religious and cultural beliefs have a substantial impact on most aspects of social behaviour. This includes the dress code, body language, expressions, speech and emotional expression. This realm of normality is not a constant phenomenon as under certain conditions it is permitted to bypass strict social codes.

Under different conditions, the social definition of normality changes even within the same group. Age, gender, social class and vocation may determine what is acceptable for one group and not for another. Within a community what is accepted as normal for one social group may be unacceptable for another. While dealing with Indo-Asians it is important to realise that a given psychiatric illness may have a different presentation in different ethnic groups and a symptom in one culture may have a different interpretation in another. For example, in Indo-Asian patients schizophrenic symptoms may be produced as a stress reaction and, in females, hallucinations are more likely to be secondary to hysteria rather than schizophrenia. For a practitioner unfamiliar with Indo-Asian customs, bizarre behaviour in an Asian elder may raise suspicion of underlying psychiatric illness but the behaviour would be acceptable to his family and to a doctor familiar with his cultural norms. All health professionals dealing with elders of Indo-Asian background should be aware of these issues. It is also important to remember, when dealing with deprived communities, that disadvantages could be erroneously labelled as psychiatric disorders.

Indo-Asian patients dislike too many questions and a long list of questions from the doctor could be construed as lack of wisdom. It may appear that the practitioner does not know the diagnosis. This is in contrast to the psychiatric work-up in the UK where interviews are conducted to extract a whole host of information about the patient, his family and the background of the symptoms. Giving a clear reason for a lengthy interview may help the patient to understand what is required and will increase their confidence in their medical practitioner.

There is some agreement on the fact that there are certain universally acceptable forms of abnormal behaviour, evidence of which could be found in practically every society. These pathologies may be given different labels in different societies and their clinical presentation may be governed by local practices.

Little research has been conducted with ethnic elders in the UK. A full review of all aspects of psychogeriatric medicine is beyond the scope of this book but a few important aspects will be described in relation to elders of Indo-Asian origin.

Indo-Asians and psychiatric illness

Primarily based upon their experiences on the Indian subcontinent, most Indo-Asians have a very low opinion of psychiatry and psychiatric illnesses. In the main, psychiatric care for the general public in South East Asia is appalling. With a few exceptions, most psychiatric hospitals are dreaded by the public and patients are admitted to these institutions only as a last resort. Big Victorian-style psychiatric hospitals are still operational but the psychiatric care in these institutions is rudimentary and primitive.

Psychiatric illnesses raise more concern in Indo-Asians than any physical pathology. There are social taboos attached to mental disorders, which can affect the social standing of the whole family. There is a generally held belief that mental disorders have a genetic basis and run in families. Business dealings, social interaction and particularly marriage prospects can be adversely affected for several generations.

Supernatural influences

Most Indo-Asians would try and give an alternative supernatural explanation for mental illness. Black magic, demonic possession, ghosts, spirits, the evil eye and poison can be cited. Many illnesses, for example epilepsy or schizophrenia, are still considered to be due to demonic possession. It is common practice in rural areas to put a shoe near a fitting patient's nose to exorcise evil spirits. Once the patient stops fitting in the post-ictal phase, the shoe is removed and the patient is declared free of evil spirits. These concepts are commonly observed in migrants from rural communities of the Indian subcontinent. Though more common in the lower socio-economic migrant groups in the UK, they may be seen in the middle classes and professional sections of the community.

Religious beliefs

People go to religious healers *(pirs)* or faith healers, who do not regurgitate scientific jargon but talk to people in their own language, with ideas they are familiar with. Nearly everyone around the world can understand the concept of magic, demons, ghosts and spirits, irrespective of their religious or social status. These concepts have been part of all cultures for centuries. Hence it is easier to 'understand' the problem and blame demons or ghosts for apocalyptic phenomena or unexplained illness. Consulting *pirs* or faith healers is quite acceptable in these societies and there are no social taboos attached to the diagnosis of black magic or demonic possession.

Protective charms (taveez)

The *taveez* is a protective charm which is worn suspended usually by a black cord around the neck, encased in either a leather or miniature silver alloy box. Occasionally it is tied over the biceps muscle around the upper arm. The casing contains a piece of paper with either religious or in some cases non-religious inscriptions or writings. Commonly seen on Muslims, a *taveez* is supposed to protect the person wearing it from the evil eye, black magic or ill will. The *taveez* could be given as a protection against an illness and hence should not be removed when patients come to hospital. Any such move without explanation would cause extreme distress and anxiety to the patient and their relatives. Some patients wear a thread instead of a *taveez* but the reason for wearing it is the same. Threads or cords can be seen in both Muslim and non-Muslim patients. Wearing stones and crystals with special protective powers is also common in Indo-Asian elders and some will be seen wearing several finger rings with different stones.

Many spiritual and faith healers do not prescribe medicine but claim to treat illness by religious texts and protective charms of various sorts. They believe that each verse of religious text has supernatural powers and provides protection against ailments as well as social evils. Spiritual healers are common in all Indo-Asian communities and protective charms are readily available all over the UK.

Somatisation

Medicine practised in the Western world primarily uses the evidence-based model. Subjective symptoms are taken seriously only when there are objective signs, backed by investigations providing scientific evidence, for a disease process. Hence health may be defined as a state of well-being within certain parameters of diagnostic technology and in the absence of objective clinical signs of disease. This model focuses on the physical dimensions of health and takes less notice of the cultural and psychological dimensions.

Somatisation is the expression of psychological symptoms via physical symptoms and signs. It is fairly common in elders of Indo-Asian origin especially when there are language barriers. There is evidence that immigrants often manifest depression in the form of somatic symptoms such as generalised weakness and non-specific aches and pains. Somatisation may represent a culturally acceptable way of expressing personal suffering, anxiety and despondency. Pain may replace the verbal expression of depression for the word 'depression', as used in the West, does not exist in many Indo-Asian languages. This is more common in the lower socio-economic classes where exposure to Western influences is less prevalent. In the middle and professional classes, fully integrated with Western philosophy, it is relatively uncommon. However, this is a generalisation and one should avoid overemphasis on these characteristics.

In most cases the somatisation presents as non-specific and vague symptoms but in certain cultures the symptoms refer to a single organ or a physiological system such as the abdomen or lower gastrointestinal tract. The organ or the system usually has a symbolic significance within that culture. One of the prime examples is seen in many North Indian Punjabi and Pakistani communities where an expression of cardiac symptoms is common. This phenomenon is labelled cultural somatisation.

There are other expressions of distress which, though closely related to somatisation, have less emphasis on physical symptoms. These may just be expressions of discontent or extreme unhappiness and are usually specific to certain cultures and communities.

It is important to be aware of the patterns of somatisation and expressions commonly used by Indo-Asian elders to communicate feelings such as anxiety and depression. An insight into these phenomena is vital in dealing with such elders.

Depression

Depression is common all over the world and particularly so in old age, mainly in those who have concurrent physical illness. The incidence of this disorder is increasing and in future, it is likely to be one of the commonest causes for disability worldwide.

Depression is often missed or ignored, particularly in the elderly in whom several physical illnesses co-exist. Its incidence ranges from around 11% in the community and 20% in institutionalised patients to nearly 45% in hospitalised elderly patients. Female sex, poor socio-economic group and the very elderly seem to be most at risk. Patients with stroke, Parkinson's disease and debilitating chronic illnesses are more commonly affected. Poverty, bereavement and social isolation are the main social factors.

Depression is easy to diagnose when it presents with classic features but in old age the presentation may be less obvious. Older people present more commonly with somatic symptoms. Suicidal ideas are common and should be taken very seriously. In these patients, cognitive impairment and depression go hand in hand and cause major diagnostic problems. Therefore depression is one of the main differential diagnoses in treating patients with dementia. Rating scales are of use in differentiating dementia from depression but this is a difficult area which needs expert advice.

Treatment of depression in old age is mainly with antidepressants but there are increased side effects, including the increased propensity to fall. Psychotherapy is underused in the elderly but is more effective if combined with antidepressants. Electroconvulsive therapy is rarely used in the elderly and is reserved for severe or resistant depression.

Prognosis of depression in old age is no different from that in younger patients but factors that are associated with poor outcome are more common in old age. These factors include concurrent physical illness, cognitive impairment, disability and severe depression at the onset. The prognosis is worse in older women than men. Maintenance antidepressant therapy is useful in preventing relapses and in most elderly patients long-term therapy is prescribed.

There are few studies which explore depression in elders of Indo-Asian origin. Psychiatric problems are considered taboo in all Indo-Asian communities and the families may go a long way to hide them. Depression is not a familiar diagnosis to elders from the Indian subcontinent. It is seen mainly as a disease of Western countries and there are no words to describe it in some South East Asian languages such as Punjabi.

Anecdotal evidence suggests that depression is common in elders of Indo-Asian origin living in the UK. More information is desperately needed to explore psychiatric problems in this group.

Suicide

There is evidence that migration increases stresses and in some migrant populations there is increased risk of suicide. This is not the case in Indo-Asians. Suicide is uncommon in Indo-Asian elders as it is prohibited by religion in most groups. However, studies have shown that though the rate of suicide in the Indian, Bangladeshi and Pakistani populations living in the UK was lower than the native population, their rate was higher than that in their countries of origin. This was true especially for females. These studies included people of all ages and were not reflective of trends in the older population.

Substance abuse

Substance abuse in the Indo-Asian elderly is very rare though there are no research data to support this view. Several substances are commonly used in the Indian subcontinent but the two important ones are cannabis and opium. Although their possession or use is illegal in the UK, health professionals working with the Indo-Asian community should have knowledge of the names, properties and symptoms of intoxication.

Cannabis (charras)

Cannabis intoxication produces acute schizophrenia, hallucinations, paranoia, excitement or an acute confusional state. It is readily available all over the Indian subcontinent where its use is not confined to any age group. It is commonly smoked and is known as *charras*. Being cheap, its use is common in the underprivileged classes both in rural areas as well as the cities. Cannabis when consumed orally is called *bhang*. It is sometimes mixed with food products such as poppadum or onion bhaji or mixed with drinks. This mode of cannabis use is seen more during festivals and times of celebration. Overall, cannabis intake is not widely acceptable in the Indo-Asian community in the

UK. Chronic abuse of cannabis can lead to a state of indolent withdrawal similar to the state seen in patients with chronic schizophrenia.

Opium (affem)

Commonly known as *affem*, the use of opium has been part of many cultures for centuries. Available all over the Indian subcontinent, it is cheap and hence abused by lower socio-economic classes. Its use is not restricted to any one age group. Chronic abuse is not uncommon.

Other drugs

Abuse of synthetic hallucinogens and cocaine is more common in affluent communities and younger age groups. Their use is less common in the Indian subcontinent and as they are relatively new to Indo-Asian culture, the elderly may not be as familiar with these substances.

Cultural syndromes

In every culture there are some specific disorders which are difficult to classify. There is no scientific basis for symptoms and no evidence exists for an organic pathology. However, the patient remains convinced of the presence of a specific pathology. One such syndrome is commonly seen in India where it is called *dhat* and in Pakistan where it is known as *jaryan*. Male patients have a firm belief that they lose sperm in their urine. Wastage of sperm in this manner is synonymous with loss of vitality and strength and hence induces extreme stress in these patients. The syndrome can be encountered in any age group and may be given as an explanation for poor health.

Dementia

There is very little scientific information available on the incidence of dementia in Indo-Asian elders. There may be an increase in vascular dementia in this population as there is increased incidence of cardiovascular pathology, diabetes and stroke. However, data are lacking on the incidence of Alzheimer's disease in Indo-Asian elders residing in the UK.

Migration and stress

The stresses of migration are well described and affect all immigrants no matter what their background. The nature of the stresses may differ from an asylum seeker to an economic migrant but for many Indo-Asians, stresses manifest in similar ways.

Refugees constitute a unique group and merit special consideration in respect of psychiatric problems. Refugees are forced to flee their countries due to conflict, wars, natural calamities and other insufferable conditions. The migratory period may be short, leaving little time to readjust. The initial shock from the disaster and trauma of leaving the homeland plus the sudden change to an alien culture compounded with all the stresses of migration can lead to a high incidence of psychiatric problems.

Economic migrants, on the other hand, have to deal with different kinds of stress. Working abroad, they are supporting their families back home as well as contributing to the economies of both the host country and that of their country of origin. Their contributions to their native and host countries have generally been ignored. Little has been done to solve their problems and regularise the system. There is a strong need to devise policies for protecting and facilitating individual migrants and their families. There are benefits to be achieved for all.

An Indo-Asian immigrant has to make many adjustments to their lifestyle following their arrival in the UK. These adjustments and changes may appear trivial but can lead to increased stress, particularly for older people. The ability to deal with change decreases with age and cultural habits set for decades may not be amenable to sudden modification.

Even elders of Indo-Asian origin who have lived in the UK for some time suffer from the stress of migration despite being resident in this country for decades. They are subject to seemingly endless changes, anything from change in clothing to personal hygiene. They are also confronted with an alien ideology of personal independence and individualism, in strong contrast to their native cultures where family and community take priority over individual preferences. Many Indo-Asian elders are used to a warmer, more predictable climate where many domestic and social activities are conducted outdoors. The unpredictable nature of the weather and change in housing may result in their being cooped up in small inner-city houses with far less social contact with the outside community.

The language barrier leads to more stress than any other factor. Inability to communicate leads to social isolation, lack of independence and inability to develop relationships. Life on the whole in the UK is more isolated for elders as compared with the Indian subcontinent. Poor command of language in the host country exaggerates these problems even further.

The elderly exile

The dream of one day returning to the homeland is very much alive in the hearts and minds of many Indo-Asian elders. After securing financial independence and fulfilling social and domestic responsibilities, they see retirement as the time to return to the motherland with pride and joy. For many this dream keeps them afloat during the years of hardship. Many elders came as economic migrants and never intended to settle in the host country.

Following retirement and at the start of old age, for the first time they confront the fact that the option of returning to their homeland is no longer available. In some cases there is no one left in the home country to return to, as all the friends and relatives have either passed away or moved to other countries. In other cases changes in social and political structure in the home country make it less attractive for them to return. There are a few unlucky ones who for medical reasons are not able to travel or are frightened to visit their homelands where modern medical facilities are not available. There is also their attachment to their immediate family, especially children and grandchildren, who consider themselves British and therefore may be unwilling to uproot themselves. It dawns upon the elders that they are no longer migrant workers but settlers and this reality can induce anxiety or depression.

There is ample evidence that immigrants have a higher incidence of psychiatric illness as compared with the native population. The incidence of psychiatric illness is also higher for immigrants as compared with people of the same ethnic background born in the host country.

Conclusion

There is little information on psychiatric problems in Indo-Asian elders. Major deficiencies exist in the recognition of their psychiatric needs and the provision of psychiatric services. The burden of psychiatric illness not only affects the patient but places overwhelming responsibilities on their families, friends and carers. Recognition and early treatment may reduce illness and dependency in many elderly people who might otherwise suffer in silence.

Further reading

Burke AW (1976) Attempted suicide among Asian immigrants in Birmingham. *Br J Psychiatr.* **128**: 528–33.

Helman CG (2000) *Culture, Health and Illness.* Butterworth Heinemann, Oxford.

Henley A and Schott J (2002) *Culture, Religion and Patient Care in a Multi-Ethnic Society.* Age Concern, London.

Institute of Medicine (2001) *Neurological, Psychiatric, and Developmental Disorders: meeting the challenge in the developing world.* National Academy Press, Washington, DC.

Murray C and Lopez A (1996) *The Global Burden of Diseases: a comprehensive assessment of mortality and disability from diseases, injuries and risk factors in 1990 and projected to 2020.* Harvard School of Public Health, WHO, and World Bank, Boston.

Rack P (1993) *Race, Culture and Mental Disorder.* Routledge, London.

Chapter 11

Death and bereavement among Indo-Asians

Introduction

There are special needs in every Indo-Asian community in coping with death and bereavement and abiding by particular religious rituals and beliefs. We have tried to summarise these needs by consulting religious leaders, using personal experiences and checking available literature.

Table 11.1 Information on country of origin and religion

	Muslims	Hindus	Sikhs	Buddhists	Christians
Main country of origin	Pakistan, Bangladesh	India, Nepal, Sri Lanka, West Indies, East Africa	India, East Africa	Sri Lanka	India, West Indies
Religious belief	Islam Monotheism	Hinduism Polytheism	Sikhism Monotheism	Buddism Monotheism	Christanity Monotheism
Reincarnation	No	Yes	Yes	Yes	No
Place of worship	Mosque	Temple	*Gurdwara*	Temple	Church
Religious leaders	Imam	Poojari	Priest	Priest	Priest
Scripture	*Koran*	*Bhagavat Gita*	*Sri Guru Granth Sahib*	Pali canon	Old & New Testament
Population in the UK	1 591 417	558 810	336 149	151 816	Under 30 000
Method of disposal of body	Burial	Cremation	Cremation	Cremation	Burial or cremation

Procedures and practice at death

Islam

Islam, which means 'surrender to God's will', is the Arabic name for the Muslim and includes the acceptance of commands and ordinances of the Prophet Mohammed. Mecca is the religious centre and a place of pilgrimage and *The Koran* is the scripture. There are five pillars of Islam.

1 Praying five times a day.
2 Giving alms.
3 Fasting during Ramadan.
4 *Zakat* or giving charity to the needy.
5 *Hajj,* pilgrimage to Mecca at least once.

Care of the dying

- Some Muslim patients may express a wish to die at home.
- The dying patient may wish to face towards Mecca.
- Relatives and friends are traditionally bound to visit the dying patient. This may cause difficulties when nursing staff resist frequent visits by family and friends.
- Muslims traditionally like to recite prayers from *The Koran* near the dying person. Sometimes an imam or a mullah may recite prayers close to the dying person's ear, usually when the patient is moribund.
- If no relatives are available, any practising Muslim can give religious comfort and advice should be sought from the local mosque and imam.

Procedure for preparing the body

- The body should not be touched by a non-Muslim. Health workers must consult the family before arranging any procedure and wear disposable gloves.
- Remove all lines and drains.
- Close the eyes and bandage the jaw so the mouth does not gape.
- Tie the feet together with a bandage around the toes.
- Straighten the body immediately after death. This will facilitate washing and shrouding the body.
- Turn the head towards the right side so that the head faces towards Mecca when the body is buried.
- Many families would like to perform the above procedures themselves.
- Do not wash the body or cut nails, scalp hair or beard.
- Cover with a white sheet.
- Muslims are buried and not cremated. The funeral should take place as soon as possible, preferably within 24 hours.
- Contact the family or the local Muslim community if family is not available.

Post-mortem and organ donation

- In Islam, the body is considered to belong to God so post-mortems are prohibited. Hence post-mortem examination is *haraam*, meaning forbidden, if carried out for educational purposes on a Muslim. Post-mortem for determination of the cause of death under the law of the land is permissible. Families will resist any request for a post-mortem unless ordered by a coroner. Reasons for a post-mortem should be explained clearly and with sensitivity.
- Embalming the body is prohibited unless required by law when sent overseas for burial.
- Organ donation is a sensitive issue and is generally not authorised by the families. There is some conflict on this issue between Muslim scholars. Some *ulema* (scholars) have dissented, citing that the human body is *amaanat* (for safe keeping) and cannot be tampered with. However, some agree that Islam

does not forbid outright cadaver organ donation. This subject should not be raised unless initiated by the family.

Notification to the coroner

- The duty inspector at the local police station should be contacted and told the deceased is a Muslim. The duty inspector will have a list of the coroner's officers who will be on call. The coroner's officer will communicate with the doctor in charge and the family.
- If a post-mortem is carried out the funeral may be delayed.
- Post-mortem can be arranged on the day or next morning and the report may be available to the coroner by telephone.
- The death certificate can be issued as soon as possible for burial within 24 hours.

Table 11.2 Information which may be helpful when dealing with a dying Muslim patient

	Address	Telephone number
Local mosque		
Funeral directors		
Burial grounds used by the local Muslim community		
Local imam		

Traditionally Muslim families do not eat until the body is buried. This may not always be possible in the UK. Friends and relatives provide food for the first three days of official mourning. Most families exercise self-discipline and avoid showing grief in public but loud wailing is still observed by some communities.

Hinduism

Hindus originate from India, Nepal, Sri Lanka (Tamils), East Africa and the West Indies. Hindus believe in one God who is worshipped in many different forms. In practice it is a polytheistic religion influenced by local cultural and social structures. Different Hindu communities have different methods of expressing their faith and practising their rituals in their own local temples. They exhibit great tolerance for other people's beliefs, revere the old and offer hospitality to any visitors. They believe in reincarnation and the caste system. Most Hindu homes will have a holy shrine. The scripture is the *Bhagavat Gita*.

Care of the dying:

- A devout Hindu who is terminally ill may receive comfort from listening to hymns and chanting from the *Bhagavat Gita*.
- A Hindu priest (*poojari*) gives the last rites. He usually comes from the local temple and is invited by the family. If there is no family he could be asked to come if the patient wishes.
- The priest may tie a thread around the patient's neck or wrist while chanting Sanskrit hymns.
- He may sprinkle or put holy Ganges water and *tulsi* (basal) leaf in the patient's mouth.
- Some patient may wish to die at home.

Procedure for preparing the body

- The funeral should take place as soon as possible. In India the funeral takes place within 24 hours but in the UK it might take several days because of protocols and pressures on the crematorium services.
- The family will wish to wash the body and conduct funeral rituals at home.
- In hospital the nurse must wear disposable gloves while preparing the body The eyes must be closed and the limbs straightened.
- Sacred threads, jewellery and other religious objects should *not* be removed.
- Wrap the body in a plain sheet. Do not add any religious emblems or wash the body.
- Adult Hindus are cremated, whereas infants and young children are buried.

Post-mortem and organ donation

There are no religious objections to organ donation but these practices are disliked.

Notification to the coroner

- Any reason for referring to the coroner should be carefully explained, if necessary with the help of an interpreter.
- Ritual preparation of the body can commence after the post-mortem.

Table 11.3 information which may be helpful when dealing with a dying Hindu patient

	Address	Telephone number
Local temple		
Funeral directors		
Local *poojari* (priest)		
Preferred crematoria		

Buddhism

Buddhism takes its name from the title 'Buddha' (the Enlightened One) which was given to the prophet Lord Guatama who lived in the Himalayan kingdom of present-day Nepal. Buddhism spread beyond India to Sri Lanka, Myanmar (Burma), Tibet, China, Japan, Korea, Vietnam and the Philippines. In the UK, apart from the Indo-Asian Buddhists, there is a big population of native converts.

The Buddhist faith centres on the teachings of Buddha and the example of how he lived his life. He is not seen as a god though his idol is worshipped in shrines. The act of *puja* (worship), which includes chanting, is the way of acknowledging the ideals set by Buddha. Buddhists believe in reincarnation and *karma*, the belief that one's actions in this current life may have consequences in subsequent lives. So individuals must behave properly and not harm or kill. There are three different denominations of Buddhism in the UK.

Care of the dying

A peaceful state of mind at the time of death is paramount. To achieve this, the dying patient and their relatives may seek help from fellow Buddhists and the priest. The Buddhist priest and relatives may chant Buddhist *slokas* (hymns) to the dying patient.

Procedure for preparing the body

- There are no formal or ritual requirements for preparing the body.
- Inform the local Buddhist priest or monk, ideally from the same denomination.
- Cremation is practised.

Table 11.4 Information which may be helpful when dealing with a dying Buddhist patient

	Address	Telephone number
Local temple		
Local priest or monk		
Funeral director		
Preferred crematorium		

Sikhism

The Sikh religion was founded by Guru Nanak in the 16th century as a reformist movement to combine the best features of Hinduism and Islam. There are 10 Sikh gurus. Guru Gobind Singh (1666–1708) established the *Khalsa Panth* of soldier-saints to defend the faith. The Khalsa men and women follow the Sikh code of conduct strictly and will adhere to the five prescribed physical articles of faith, the *five Ks*.

Table 11.5 The *five Ks*

	Physical article	Symbolic meaning
Kesh	Uncut scalp hair and beard	Dedication and group consciousness
Kirpan	Ceremonial sword	Struggle against injustice
Kangha	Comb in hair	Hygiene and discipline
Kara	Steel bracelet worn on right wrist	Restraint in their actions
Kachha	Short pants or undergarment	Self-control and chastity

The turban (*dastar*) is also important, symbolising royalty and dignity. The scripture is the *Sri Guru Granth Sahib*.

Care of the dying

A terminally ill Sikh patient may receive comfort from hearing hymns from the *Sri Guru Granth Sahib* recited by a priest from the Sikh Gurdwara (temple), a relative or a friend.

Procedure for preparing the body

- The family will be responsible for all the rites and rituals such as washing and laying out of the body.
- Special regard must be given to the five Ks. Scalp hair and beard (*kesh*) *must not* be cut for any reason. The *kanga, kara, kirpan* and *kachha* must not be removed.
- The face must be cleaned and the eyes and mouth closed.
- The limbs are straightened and the body covered in a plain sheet or shroud without any religious emblems.
- In India adults are always cremated within 24 hours. In the UK cremation should take place as soon as possible. Sikhs are cremated wearing the five symbols of faith (the five Ks).
- Stillborn babies and neonates may be buried.

Post-mortem and organ donation

- Respect the five Ks when doing a post-mortem.
- There is no religious objection to organ transplant but it is disliked.

Notification to the coroner

Referral to the coroner must be carefully explained, if necessary with the help of an interpreter.

Table 11.6 Information which may be helpful when dealing with a dying Sikh patient

	Address	Telephone number
Local *gurdwara* (temple)		
Local priest		
Funeral director		
Preferred crematorium		

Funerals abroad

Some families may wish to take the body of the deceased to their country of origin for burial and occasionally for cremation. The family must do the following.

*   Contact a funeral director and make known their wish to take the body home to the country of origin.
*   Register the death and inform the Registrar of their intention to take the body. The Registrar will issue a copy of the death certificate for the family to give to the funeral director. There is a fee for this service.

The funeral director will arrange the following.

*   Apply to the coroner for an 'out of England order' which is granted within a day or so.
*   Apply to the airline which will carry the body. Pakistan Airways, Bangladesh Biman, Air India, Air Lanka and British Airways are the usual carriers.
*   A 'freedom of infection' certificate must be obtained from the doctor who originally issued the death certificate. This is to confirm that the patient did not die of any infectious disease. There will be a standard fee charged by the doctor.
*   The body is carried in a zinc-lined coffin which is hermetically sealed.
*   A certificate to confirm that the body has been embalmed may be necessary.
*   Some countries of origin will require a consular seal from the relevant embassy or High Commission.
*   The funeral director will organise all transport arrangements.

If death is due to unnatural causes, such as homicide, repatriation of the body will not be allowed until the court proceedings are complete.

Patterns of mortality

Some studies have shown different patterns of mortality in migrants from the Indian subcontinent. Some diseases exceeded expected mortality in this community and these included deaths from infection, diabetes, ischaemic heart disease and cirrhosis. Deaths from malignant diseases were less notable but included bronchogenic carcinoma.

Information on patterns of mortality in various ethnic groups is lacking. There is the possibility of gaining more information and insight into the health needs of Indo-Asians by mapping patterns of mortality in these groups.

Further reading

Balarajan R (1997) Patterns of mortality among Sri Lankans in England and Wales. *Health Trends*. **29**: 3–6.

Balarajan R, Bulusu L, Adelstein AM and Shukla V (1984) Pattern of mortality among migrants to England and Wales from the Indian subcontinent. *BMJ.* **289**: 1185–7.

Helman CG (2000) *Culture, Health and Illness.* Butterworth Heinemann, Oxford.

Henley A and Schott J (2002) *Culture, Religion and Patient Care in a Multi-Ethnic Society.* Age Concern, London.

Chapter 12

Alternative medicine and Indo-Asian elders

Introduction

Alternative medicine is a broad subject and includes all modalities of medical management or treatment other than those provided by orthodox Western medicine.

Each group of migrants brings with it its traditions, culture and, of course, its brand of traditional medicine. To provide adequate healthcare, health professionals need to have an understanding of alternative medicine practised in the community.

On the Indian subcontinent traditional medicine plays a major role in the healthcare needs of the general population. Being widely available and considerably cheaper than orthodox Western medicine, it is not surprising that the vast majority of the population use alternative medicine as their principal health provider. Traditional medicine is widely popular in all sections of society and enjoys support from governments in the region. The providers of traditional healthcare outnumber doctors in these countries by a large margin. In many rural areas these practitioners are the only available health providers. Many of these practitioners are trained by their own colleges and are registered with their parent organisations. They have their own pharmaceutical industries which produce large number of products, many available in Asian supermarkets in the UK. Many are sold over the counter or are available by mail order.

The two most commonly practised systems of traditional alternative medicine are Ayurveda and Tibb-i-Unnani. Both systems are based on the hot and cold equilibrium of the body and the ability of food and herbs to influence this balance. Although they predominantly use herbs and lay stress on food products in treatment regimens, the use of Western medicine is fairly common. The concept of 'hot' or 'cold' food bears no relationship to the temperature of the food or its taste. To an untrained eye the whole system may seem strange and arbitrary.

Ayurvedic medicine

Ayurvedic medicine is the traditional medicine of India which has been practised for thousands of years and has its own unique philosophy. It is based on the concept of balance of energies in the body. Illness occurs as a result of the imbalance of these energies. The practitioner is called a *vaid*. The treatment recognises that all human beings have different constitutions and medicine is administered according to individual needs.

Tibb-i-Unnani

Tibb-i-Unnani or *hikmat* was developed by the Arabs from their traditional medicine but its roots go back as far as ancient Greek medicine. It is widely practised in the Indian subcontinent and the Islamic world. The practitioner is called a *hakim*. Tibb-i-Unnani is based on the concept that the body's main constituents are blood, phlegm, yellow bile and black bile. They have the characteristics of being hot, cold, wet or dry. An illness could be secondary to any of these characteristics, for example it could be due to excess cold, heat, dryness or wetness in the body. Restoring this balance could rectify the illness.

The *hakim* mainly makes the diagnosis by feeling the pulse at the wrist with two fingers. The right radial pulse is felt in males and the left in females. Illnesses are treated by giving extensive advice on relevant food products in an effort to help the patient restore their equilibrium. Nearly every patient will be given a potion produced by the *hakim* and consisting mainly of herbs and plant products.

For centuries, it has been standard practice for the *hakim* to prescribe *kushtas*, mainly for sexual problems, many as aphrodisiacs. These contain potentially toxic oxidised heavy metals such as mercury, gold, arsenic, lead, silver and gold. These products, which are now illegal, could cause heavy metal poisoning and are responsible for chronic ill health in some patients.

Hakims are well versed in the local customs and are respected members of the community. Providing a counselling service is an important part of their clinical practice and the community consults them on many non-medical matters. Being at the heart of the community is the key factor in the *hakim's* success.

Homeopathy

Practised for nearly 200 years, homeopathy claims to treat by stimulating the body to heal itself. This form of alternative medicine is widely popular in the Indian subcontinent. As it is considered safer than many other forms of alternative medicine, many prefer it along with orthodox Western medicine.

Indo-Asian elders and alternative medicine

Many elders of Indo-Asian origin still consult *hakims* or *vaids*. Research shows that many problems referred to these practitioners are either psychiatric or psychosexual. Problems related to the digestive tract and non-specific illnesses are also commonly treated by *hakims* or *vaids*. Elderly people are more familiar with alternative medicine in their countries of origin and hence more likely to use it in the UK, along with orthodox Western medicine. Many would consult their general practitioner first or a hospital physician. The alternative medicine is used mainly as an adjunct and often after orthodox Western medicine has been unable to relieve them of their problem. One should bear in mind that many patients, if confronted, would deny use of alternative medicine to their doctors or health professionals as they fear that this might offend them.

Being accustomed to *hakims* or *vaids*, many Indo-Asian patients may not like to be asked too many questions. The philosophy of alternative medicine is to provide a diagnosis or an explanation along with hope and comfort. This is in contrast to a conventional medical work-up where interviews are conducted to extract a whole host of information about the patient, his family and the background of the symptoms. A battery of investigations is followed by several visits to hospitals where patients are unlikely to see the same doctor twice. Some patients are left without a clear explanation of their symptoms or illness. This understandably leads to loss of confidence in Western medicine.

Religious healers

Religious healers are seen in practically every Indo-Asian community. They traditionally do not prescribe medications and claim to heal by the use of religious scripts. They may be part of the community but going to the religious healer of another community is not uncommon.

The evil eye or *nazar* is not a concept unique to Indo-Asians. Many Indo-Asians, especially the elderly, firmly believe in the power of the evil eye. The problems caused by *nazar* are usually minor and not life threatening. The religious healer is the most likely person to be consulted for an ailment if it were considered to caused by the evil eye.

A *taveez* (*see* Chapter 10) is a protective charm, which is usually given by a religious healer. Most commonly seen in Muslims, a *taveez* is supposed to heal an illness or protect the person from the evil eye, black magic or ill will.

Spiritual healers

Similar to religious healers, these practitioners differ in the sense that they do not observe barriers of race or religion. They do not prescribe medicine and claim to cure by the supernatural powers or gifts they possess. Many advertise their services in the local newspapers.

Conclusion

The use of alternative medicine by Indo-Asian elders in the UK is unlikely to change in the foreseeable future. Despite adverse publicity, many people favour these modalities of treatment. Knowledge of and familiarity with types of alternative medicine used by the local community are important for health providers.

Chapter 13

Commonly encountered medical problems

In the UK there are a few medical conditions which are more common in Indo-Asians compared with the Caucasian population. Awareness of these pathologies is important when dealing with Indo-Asian elders.

Renal disease

There is clear evidence that Indo-Asians have higher susceptibility to renal disease as compared with the Caucasian population. Diabetics have a high incidence of renal failure but in the Indo-Asian population without diabetes, the risk of developing end-stage renal failure is three-fold higher than in the native population. An increased incidence of obesity, hypertension and cardiovascular disease may play some part in this predisposition.

There are no studies linking the increased susceptibility to renal disease with genetic factors but there is an increased incidence of renal disease in first-degree relatives. Intrauterine growth retardation, foetal malnutrition, low birth weight, thrifty genotype and thrifty phenotype have all been postulated as possible explanations for the increased propensity to renal disease in Indo-Asians. Detailed information on thrifty genotype and thrifty phenotype has been given in Chapter 5.

Type 2 diabetes

Nearly a quarter of Indo-Asian elders suffer from Type 2 diabetes. In some studies 40% of Indo-Asians presenting with end-stage renal failure had diabetes as compared with the white population where only 20% had Type 2 diabetes. Type 2 diabetes is one of the major causes of increased susceptibility to renal disease. The risk of Indo-Asians with diabetes developing end-stage renal failure is 13 times that of the white population.

Other causes

Indo-Asians have an increased prevalence of renal involvement with systemic disease such as systemic lupus. There are several other causes for the increased incidence of end-stage renal failure, including reflux nephropathy, most types of glomerulonephritis and tuberculosis. In many cases it is not possible to determine the cause of renal disease, as there is advanced disease at the time of presentation.

Renal replacement therapy and renal transplant

The experience in Leicester has provided insight into issues surrounding renal replacement therapy in Indo-Asians. Recent reports suggest that there is no difference between the white population and Indo-Asians as far as infection or complication-free survival is concerned. Neither is there any difference in graft survival for cadaveric renal transplant. However, inequalities of access to cadaveric transplant exist for the Indo-Asian population. This may be because organ donation in Indo-Asians is particularly low.

End-stage renal disease is increasing in Indo-Asian elders at an alarming rate. Inequalities of health access and referral to specialised services have been raised as problem areas. Late referral for the first presentation is associated with increased morbidity and mortality. Accelerated cardiovascular disease is the most important cause of death in patients with end-stage renal failure. A holistic approach is required in these patients with emphasis on changes in lifestyle and control of risk factors. Screening and early intervention have their merits if applied appropriately to high-risk communities and Indo-Asians elders may be an ideal group for such intervention. Living donors for renal transplant should be encouraged and communities need to review the reasons for low cadaveric organ donation.

Haematological disorders

Anaemia

Anaemia is not uncommon in the Indo-Asian community and has several aetiologies.

Iron deficiency anaemia is common but its prevalence in Indo-Asian elders is not known. Vegetarian diet or poor diet for economic reasons may contribute to this pathology. Hookworm infection is very common in the Indian subcontinent and should always be considered as a possibility in Indo-Asian elders, particularly when they have been visiting friends and family from their country of origin. These possibilities should be excluded by baseline tests before more invasive investigations are contemplated to exclude bowel malignancy. Mildly low haemoglobin with low mean corpuscular volume (MCV) is seen in patients with beta thalassaemia trait and can be confused with iron deficiency anaemia. These patients may have higher iron reserves and prescribing iron replacement will be futile. Beta thalassaemia is commonly seen in patients from the Indian subcontinent and the trait is not uncommon in the elderly of Indo-Asian origin.

Vitamin B12 deficiency is seen in the elderly population as a cause of chronic anaemia. Vitamin B12 is found mainly in the animal kingdom. Elders who are strict vegans and do not consume any animal products, including eggs and dairy produce, are more likely to develop B12 deficiency. Seaweed and whole wheat have some vitamin B12. Pernicious anaemia is less common in the Indo-Asian community.

Chronic anaemia may be encountered in patients with heavy metal poisoning. This could be as a result of using *surma* or *kohl* (lead poisoning) or consuming heavy metals used in alternative medicine (arsenic poisoning).

Glucose-6-phosphate dehydrogenase deficiency is also seen in people from northern India.

Osteomalacia

Osteomalacia is a defect in bone mineralisation secondary to vitamin D deficiency or its metabolism. It is only encountered in adults when the epiphyseal plates have united. The two major causes of this disorder include a diet deficient in vitamin D and inadequate exposure to sunlight. As the Asian skin is more pigmented, ultraviolet rays in sunlight are less able to penetrate and this reduces production of vitamin D by the skin. The traditional clothing worn by elders from ethnic minorities further reduces their exposure to sunlight. Women are particularly affected as traditionally they are supposed to cover most of their bodies except for the face and hands. A home-bound lifestyle and less participation in outdoor activities may also contribute to this problem. Vegetarian diet is also a contributory factor for vitamin D deficiency. Chapatti flour contributes to the development of vitamin D deficiency. First-generation immigrants, especially the elderly, are more likely to adhere to their customs and hence be more prone to vitamin D deficiency, which seems to be most severe in the Hindu population.

This diagnosis is commonly missed in elderly Asian women where the presentation may only include non-specific aches and pains. Measurement of vitamin D levels is essential in all Asian patients with non-specific aches and pains, proximal myopathy, bony tenderness and low-trauma fractures. There is an association of impaired immune functions and vitamin B12 deficiency in patients with osteomalacia. Apart from prescribing vitamin D supplements to the patient, screening the family and spouse is recommended.

Hip fractures

The true incidence of hip fracture in the Indo-Asian community and the differences between various cultural groups are unknown. There is evidence that the risk of hip fracture is higher in Indo-Asian elders. Fractures occur at an earlier age compared with the white population and the incidence of subtrochanteric fractures is higher. This pattern of hip fracture suggests underlying bone disorder in Indo-Asian elders and strengthens the possibility that the cause of hip fracture in this population may be different. Vitamin D deficiency may play an important role.

With the increase in numbers of Indo-Asian elders in the UK, there is likely to be an increase in hip fracture numbers. Rehabilitation and nursing care may be affected by language and cultural differences.

Heavy metal poisoning

Kushtas

A more detailed account of these products has been given in Chapter 12. The *kushtas*, mainly prescribed as aphrodisiacs, contain toxic oxidised heavy metals such as mercury, arsenic, lead, silver and gold. These products could cause heavy metal poisoning and could account for chronic ill health in some patients. Their effects can range from mild aches and pains, anaemia and lassitude to neuronal, cardiac and hepatic toxicity.

Surma

Surma or *kohl* is widely used by Indo-Asians of all ages as a prophylactic agent to protect eyes against disease and as a 'vision enhancer'. There are several varieties of *surma* available from Asian stores in the UK. The main component of *surma* is lead sulphide which can lead to chronic lead poisoning.

Acute abdomen

Certain pathologies should be considered when dealing with an elderly patient from the Indian subcontinent. The patient could be a visitor to the UK, a holidaymaker or a British national who has visited their homeland recently. In these patients, infections could be a possibility, especially caecal amoebiasis, typhoid ulceration, perforation or ileocaecal tuberculosis. Other pathologies worth considering include helminthiasis, hydatid cyst, malarial spleen and schistosomiasis. Early recognition may make a difference to the outcome.

Less common pathologies

Though evidence-based information is lacking, some pathologies are less commonly observed in the Indo-Asian population living in the UK. However, the presence of these pathologies should still be considered in elderly patients living in the UK. These pathologies include:

- polymyalgia rheumatic
- temporal arteritis
- Crohn's disease
- osteoarthritis of the hip
- multiple sclerosis.

Information on these issues may help staff to avoid pitfalls and delay in diagnosing medical problems accurately.

Further reading

Brandt KD, Doherty M and Lohmander LS (2000) *Osteoarthritis*. Oxford University Press, Oxford.

Calder SJ, Anderson GH, Harper WM and Gregg PJ (1994) Ethnic variation in epidemiology and rehabilitation of hip fracture. *BMJ*. **309**: 1124–5.

Ellis P and Cairns H (2001) Renal impairment in elderly patients with hypertension and diabetes. *Q J Med*. **94**: 261–5.

Feehally J (2003) Ethnicity and renal disease: questions and challenges. *Clin Med*. **3**(6): 578–82.

Iqbal SJ, Kaddam I, Wassif W, Nichol F and Walls J (1994) Continuing clinically severe vitamin D deficiency in Asian in the UK (Leicester). *Postgrad Med J*. **70**: 708–14.

Shaunak S, Colston K, Ang L, Patel S and Maxwell J (1985) Vitamin D deficiency in adult British Hindu Asians: a family disorder. *BMJ*. **291**: 1165–7.

Stephens WP, Klimiuk PS, Warrington S, Taylor JL, Berry JL and Mawer EB (1982) Observations on the natural history of vitamin D deficiency amongst Asian immigrants. *Q J Med*. **202**: 171–8.

Chapter 14

The Indian subcontinent

The term 'Indo-Asian' refers to people who originated from the Indian subcontinent. The Indian subcontinent encompasses four main countries, namely Bangladesh, India, Pakistan and Sri Lanka. To understand the cultural background of Indo-Asian immigrants, a short introduction is essential. This chapter provides the basic facts on the four main countries of the Indian subcontinent.

People's Republic of Bangladesh

Geography

Situated in southern Asia, the country borders Burma on the east and India on all other borders except the Bay of Bengal on the south. The capital is Dhaka.

The country is mostly flat but hilly in the south east. The climate is tropical in winter but hot and humid in summer. There is high rainfall and flooding during the monsoon season.

Water-borne diseases are common and air pollution is an issue in most large cities.

Population

138 448 210. The elderly, aged over 65 constitute 3.4% of the population.

Population growth rate

2.06%

Net migration rate

– 0.72 migrant(s)/1000 population.

Life expectancy

Total population: 61.33 years
Male: 61.46 years
Female: 61.2 years

Ethnic groups

Bengali 98%
Tribal groups
Non-Bengali Muslims

Religions

Muslim 83%
Hindu 16%
Other 1%

Languages

Bengali
English
Syleti

Literacy

Definition: age 15 and over can read and write
Total population: 43.1%
Male: 53.9%
Female: 31.8%

GDP per capita

Purchasing power parity – $1800

Population below poverty line

35.6%

Republic of India

Geography

India is situated in southern Asia, between Bangladesh and Burma on the east and Pakistan on the west. The Arabian Sea and the Bay of Bengal make its southern border and China is its most prominent northern neighbour. The capital is New Delhi.

The total area of India is 3 287 590 sq km and the climate varies from tropical monsoon in the south to temperate in the north.

Water-borne and infectious diseases are common. Air pollution is an issue in most large cities.

Population

1 049 700 118. Currently, India is the second most populated country in the world. The elderly over 65 constitute over 4.8% of the population.

Population growth

1.47%

Life expectancy

Total population: 63.62 years
Male: 62.92 years
Female: 64.37 years

Literacy rate

Definition: age 15 and over can read and write
Total population: 59.5%
Male: 70.2%
Female: 48.3%

Ethnic groups

Indo-Aryan 72%
Dravidian 25%
Mongolian and other 3%

Religions

Hindu 81.3%
Muslim 12%
Christian 2.3%
Sikh 1.9%
Jain, Parsi, Buddhist 2.5%

Languages

Hindi, the national language 30%
Bengali
Telugu
Marathi
Tamil
Urdu
Gujrati
Malayalam
Kannada
Oriya
Punjabi
Assamese
Kashmiri
Sindhi
Sanskrit
English is the most important national language for communication.

Population below poverty line

25%

GDP per capita

Purchasing power parity – $2600

Islamic Republic of Pakistan

Geography

Pakistan is located in South East Asia and stretches from the Arabian Sea in the south to the mountain ranges in the north. Pakistan shares its eastern border with India and its north Eastern border with China. Afghanistan is the north western neighbour and Iran is to the south west.

Pakistan has some of the most ancient historical sites in the world, dating back over 5000 years. The Indus Valley civilisation is one of the oldest in the world.

With a total area of 796 095 sq km, Pakistan is nearly four times the size of the UK. There is a flat plain in the Punjab but mountains in the north and north west, with the highest point being K2 (Mount Godwin-Austen, 8611 m), the second highest peak in the world. Pakistan has seven of the 16 tallest peaks in Asia and 40 of the world's 50 highest mountains are in Pakistan. The capital is Islamabad.

The climate is generally dry and hot but in the north it is colder and rainfall is high. Travellers should be aware of water pollution from sewage, industrial wastes and agricultural run-off. The majority of the population does not have access to clean drinking water. Air pollution is an issue in most large cities.

Population

150 694 740. Currently the sixth most populated country in the world. The elderly over 65 years constitute 4.2% of the population.

Population growth

2.01% (2003 estimate)

Life expectancy

Total population: 62.2 years
Male: 61.3 years
Female: 63.14 years

Net migration rate

–0.75 migrant(s)/1000 population.

Ethnic groups

Punjabi
Sindhi
Pathan
Baloch
Muhajir (immigrants from India in 1947)

Languages

Urdu (official) The second or third language of most Pakistanis
Punjabi 48%
Sindhi 12%
Siraiki (a Punjabi variant) 10%
Pashtu 8%
Balochi 3%
Hindko 2%
Brahui 1%
Burushaski and others 8%
English is widely used in government offices and is the political and commercial language.

Religions

Muslim 97% (Sunni 77%, Shi'a 20%)
Christian, Hindu and other 3%

Literacy rate

Definition: age 15 and over can read and write
Total population: 45.7%
Male: 59.8%
Female: 30.6%

GDP per capita

Purchasing power parity – $2000

Population below poverty line

35%

Sri Lanka

Geography

Sri Lanka is an island in the Indian Ocean south of India. The capital is Colombo.

The Sinhalese came to the island in the 6th century BC, probably from northern India. Buddhism came to the island in the third century BC. Southern Indian influence came in the 14th century with the establishment of the northern Tamil kingdom.

The country was invaded by the Portuguese in the 16th century and by the Dutch in the 17th century and it became a British colony in 1802. The country became independent in 1948 and its name changed to Sri Lanka (from Ceylon) in 1972.

The total area of the country is 65 610 sq km. The island is mostly flat plain but there are mountains in the south-central interior. The climate is tropical.

Water-borne diseases are common. There is high risk of water pollution by industrial wastes and sewage. Air pollution is an issue in most large cities.

Population

19 742 439
The elderly over 65 years constitute 6.9% of the population.

Life expectancy

Total population: 72.62 years
Male: 70.09 years
Female: 75.29 years

Ethnic groups

Sinhalese 74%
Tamil 18%
Moor 7%
Burgher, Malay and Vedda 1%

Religions

Buddhist 70%
Hindu 15%
Christian 8%
Muslim 7%

Languages

Sinhala (the national language) 74%
Tamil 18%
Other 8%
English is commonly used in government and is spoken competently by about 10% of the population.

Literacy

Definition: age 15 and over can read and write
Total population: 92.3%
Male: 94.8%
Female: 90%

Population below poverty line

22%

GDP per capita

Purchasing power parity – $3700

Chapter 15

Useful organisations and contacts

British Geriatric Society

www.bgs.org.uk
British Geriatric Society is the only association of specialist medical professionals practising geriatric medicine in the UK. The society provides valuable
information to anyone with an interest in the care of elderly people.

Age Concern

www.ageconcern.org.uk
Age Concern is an organisation for the support of all people aged over 50 years
in the UK. It provides essential services, advice on income and benefits, community care, health, housing, consumer issues and information. Over 40 fact sheets
are available on various issues. The organisation campaigns on age-related
issues and works to influence public opinion and government policy.

Age Concern Information Line: 0800 00 99 66.

Global Action on Ageing

www.globalageing.org
Global Action on Ageing is an international citizen group that works on issues
of concern to older people. It reports on older people's needs and potential
within the globalised world economy. Global Action on Ageing carries out
research on critical emerging topics and publishes the results. It distributes news
both directly, through its own publications, and through the mass media. It
maintains a presence at the United Nations headquarters in New York and
participates in major UN events and conferences.

Help Age International

www.helpage.org
A global network of not-for-profit organisations with a mission to work with
and for disadvantaged older people worldwide to achieve a lasting improvement
in the quality of their lives. The organisation is working in over 80 countries on
practical and policy issues.

International Organisation on Migration (IOM)

www.iom.int
IOM was established in 1951 as an intergovernmental organisation to resettle
European displaced persons, refugees and migrants. It has grown to become the

leading international organisation working with migrants and governments to encompass a variety of migration management activities throughout the world. Its main role is to highlight understanding of migration issues and uphold the human dignity and welfare of migrants.

Being an international organisation, it helps governments and civil societies throughout the world. Its mandate includes rapid humanitarian responses to sudden migration flows, assistance to migrants on their way to new homes and lives and facilitation of labour migration. Other areas of its operation include information and education on migration and research into all aspects of migration management worldwide.

IOM is not part of the United Nations but has close working relations with it. It has operational partnership with many international and non-governmental organisations.

Other organisations which deal with refugees include:

* Refugee Action: www.refugee-action.org
* North of England RefugeeService: www.refugee.org.uk

British Heart Foundation (BHF)

www.bhf.org.uk

Founded in 1961, this organisation has contributed enormously to the management and prevention of heart diseases in the UK and around the world. For patients with heart disease it provides support and information, and literature on prevention and treatment of heart disease is available at no cost. The BHF plays a vital role in funding education, training and research relating to heart disease. The organisation is at the forefront of helping patients with most forms of heart disease. The service is supported by booklets, fact sheets and videos, available free to health professionals, patients and carers.

British Hypertension Society (BHS)

www.bhsoc.org

Founded in 1981, the BHS is a scientific organisation which funds research into hypertension and related vascular disease. It also takes a lead in developing guidelines and dissemination of information on hypertension. It is a useful source of information for health professionals dealing with hypertension.

Blood Pressure Association (BPA)

www.bpassoc.org.uk

The Blood Pressure Association was founded in 2000 to provide vital information to the general public on issues about high blood pressure. It aims to improve understanding of high blood pressure among the general population. Information on medication, lifestyle, diet and general issues related to high blood pressure is available.

Chest, Heart and Stroke Scotland (CHSS)

www.chss.org.uk
The CHSS is a leading medical charity in Scotland which helps patients with chest, heart and stroke illness and aims to improve their quality of life. The society provides not only advice and information on medical research but support in the community.

The CHSS provides care and support throughout Scotland for patients, their families and carers.

Funding research into the prevention, diagnosis, treatment, rehabilitation and social impact of chest, heart and stroke illness is one of the organisation's main goals. Their Advice Line (0845 077 6000) offers advice from trained nurses on all aspects of chest, heart and stroke illness. This service is supported by booklets, fact sheets and videos, available free to patients and carers.

Hyperlipidaemia Education And Research Trust (HEART)

www.heartuk.org.uk
HEART UK provides important and useful information for patients with high cholesterol and also scientific research and good clinical practice for the management of hyperlipidaemia within the UK. HEART UK improves awareness of heart disease, stressing the importance of a healthy lifestyle in reducing the risk of heart disease. It provides information on the risks of heart disease to the public and health professionals.

Hearts For Life

www.heartsforlife.co.uk
This website is a useful resource that supplements advice patients and their carers receive about heart disease from their doctors. Material is based on the *National Service Framework for Coronary Heart Disease*, published by the Department of Health in March 2000.

High Blood Pressure Foundation

www.hbpf.org.uk
This organisation helps with basic understanding, assessment, treatment and public awareness of high blood pressure. Its work includes general welfare of people with high blood pressure

Diabetes UK

www.diabetes.org.uk
Diabetes UK is the operating name of the British Diabetic Association. Extensive information on all aspects of diabetes is available on this site. The information

is for general use only and is not intended to provide personal medical advice or substitute for the advice of a physician. A translation service is available in over 100 languages. To operate a translation service, telephone 0845 120 2960.

Stroke Association

www.stroke.org.uk

The Stroke Association is a charity which deals exclusively with stroke. It provides information, education and support for stroke patients, their families and carers.

The Stroke Information telephone helpline (0845 303 3100), dysphasia support service and family support service provide help to patients and their relatives. The Association funds research and distributes literature on stroke prevention, diagnosis, treatment and rehabilitation.

Alzheimer's Society

www.alzheimers.org.uk

Founded in 1979, the Alzheimer's Society provides information and education, support for carers and quality day and home care. It is the UK's leading care and research charity for people with dementia, their families and carers.

National Kidney Research Fund

www.nkrf.org.uk

The NKRF is a registered charity working to improve awareness of and research into renal disease. Its main focus is on informing and updating patients, their families and carers, the general public and health professionals about kidney and related diseases and the needs of those affected.

National Osteoporosis Society

www.nos.org.uk

Founded in 1986, the National Osteoporosis Society is a registered charity dedicated to improving the diagnosis, prevention and treatment of osteoporosis.

Electronic Medicines Compendium

www.medicines.org.uk

This is an information service for the UK public looking for medicines information. The service links to the specialist information written for healthcare professionals and the leaflets that come with the medicine. This can be an important resource for patients and their carers.

Consensus Action on Salt and Health (CASH)

www.hyp.ac.uk
This is a group of specialists concerned about the effect of salt on health and cardiovascular disease.

Sustrans

www.sustrans.org.uk
Sustrans works on practical projects that encourage people to walk, cycle or use public transport in order to reduce motor traffic and its adverse effects. It also runs the National Cycle Network.

Eldis: Ageing Populations Resource Guide

www.eldis.org
ELDIS is a gateway to information on development issues, providing free and easy access to a wide range of high-quality online resources. It provides summaries and links to online documents and a directory of websites, databases, library catalogues and useful email lists.

International Ageing

www.aoa.gov
This section of the Administration on Ageing website provides links to some of the major sources of information in governmental and non-governmental international organisations.

International Association of Gerontology

www.sfu.ca/iag
The International Association of Gerontology was founded in 1950. Its objectives are to promote research and training in the field of ageing.

International Institute on Ageing

www.inia.org
The International Institute on Ageing provides education and training in areas related to ageing. In accordance with its agreement with the UN and the government of Malta, the Institute fulfils the training needs of developing countries and facilitates the implementation of the Vienna International Plan of Action on Ageing.

Policy Research Institute on Ageing and Ethnicity (PRIAE)

www.priae.org

PRIAE is an independent charity working on ageing and ethnicity issues in Europe and the UK. The organisation focuses mainly on black and ethnic minority elders.

Moving Here

www.movinghere.org.uk

Moving Here is an organisation which deals with 200 years of history of migration to the UK. It explores, records and illustrates why people came to England and what their experiences were and continue to be. The site mainly looks at the Caribbean, Irish, Jewish and South Asian communities.

This website offers free access, for personal and educational use, to online versions of original material related to migration, including photographs, personal papers, government documents, maps and art objects, as well as a collection of sound recordings and video clips.

For more information on health, visit the following websites:

- National Health Service: www.nhs.uk
- Department of Health: www.doh.gov.uk
- Wired for Health (information on health for teachers and children): www.wiredforhealth.gov.uk
- Surgery Door: www.surgerydoor.co.uk
- Net Doctor: www.netdoctor.co.uk
- Well Aware: www.well-aware.co.uk
- Healthsites (a gateway to finding reliable health information): www.healthsites.co.uk
- Electronic Quality Information for Patients (how to find quality information on health on the internet): www.equip.nhs.uk
- National Institute for Clinical Excellence: www.nice.org.uk

For more information on changing lifestyles, visit the following websites:

- Action on Smoking and Health: www.ash.org.uk
- Quit: www.quit.org.uk
- No Smoking Day: www.nosmokingday.org.uk
- DASH diet: www.nhlbi.nih.gov

Index